Fertility and Conception

Fertility and Conception

an essential guide for childless couples

John J. Stangel, M.D.

*With a Foreword by Martin L. Stone, M.D., President of the
American College of Obstetricians and Gynecologists*

**PADDINGTON
PRESS LTD**

NEW YORK & LONDON

Library of Congress Cataloging in Publication Data
Stangel, John J   1941–
    Fertility and conception: an essential guide for childless
couples.
    Includes index.
    1. Sterility. 2. Conception. 3. Human reproduction.
4. Fertility, Human. I. Title.

RC889.S63   618.1'78   78-21642
ISBN 0 448 22979 X (U.S. and Canada only)
ISBN 0 7092 0732 8

Filmset in England by Tradespools Limited, Frome,
Somerset
Printed and bound in the United States

Designed by Patricia Pillay
Illustrations by Jennie Smith

IN THE UNITED STATES
PADDINGTON PRESS
Distributed by
GROSSET & DUNLAP

IN THE UNITED KINGDOM
PADDINGTON PRESS

IN CANADA
Distributed by
RANDOM HOUSE OF CANADA LTD.

IN SOUTHERN AFRICA
Distributed by
ERNEST STANTON (PUBLISHERS) (PTY.) LTD.

IN AUSTRALIA AND NEW ZEALAND
Distributed by
A. H. & A. W. REED

To Lois, my wife and my closest friend
and
*To my patients, who have shared their problems and feelings with me
and have taught me a great deal.*

Acknowledgments

IT WOULD BE impossible to list and thank all the people whose thoughts and work have influenced this book. To all who have contributed through their writing, research or personal communication I wish to express my appreciation. There are a few without whose specific assistance this volume would not be a reality. In this connection I wish to thank Richard Resnick, M.D., Walter L. Freedman, M.D., J. Victor Reyniak, M.D., Harry Settles, PhD., Carlton Eddy, PhD., Sidney Shulman, PhD., and Linsey Levine. I want to express my appreciation to Jeanne Lolya for preparing the typed manuscript. Finally I wish to thank my wife Lois for constant patience, encouragement and support.

J.J.S.

Contents

Foreword

This very timely book deals with infertility, its causes, diagnosis and treatment. It is up to date and current in covering the field at a time when new directions are being charted daily.

The author, who is quite knowledgeable and experienced, has produced a readable text for the non-professional. With skill he blends an unusual sensitivity and understanding of his patients and their needs with the scientific advances occurring so rapidly.

The format is innovative and interesting, the diagrams clear and most helpful. The result is an unusually complete and extensive text that is still easy to follow and understand. Dr. Stangel covers not only the mechanistic approaches used to investigate and treat the infertile couple but also the role of life-style factors such as stress and exercise. The latest research developments are thoroughly covered, and their implications discussed.

This excellent book will be of real value to the couple who has an infertility problem and to their physician, since their understanding of the problem will make the doctor's efforts to help more productive. Even those who have no reproductive problems will find this an informative and useful text.

MARTIN L. STONE, M.D.,
Professor and Chairman,
Department of Obstetrics and Gynecology,
State University of New York at Stony Brook, and
President of the American College of
Obstetricians and Gynecologists (1979)

Introduction

I SAT BEHIND MY DESK on a bright, spring afternoon. A woman in her late twenties sat across from me, shifted in her seat and continued talking. "I am tired of trying for something that other people take for granted. My friends are all getting pregnant and I'm not. Many of the women on my street are pregnant for the third and fourth time because they have nothing better to do, and I can't do it even once. I feel resentful when I walk down the street and see other women pushing baby carriages. Jeff and I have tried for so long that I just can't stand it any longer. Sex used to be one of the most enjoyable things in our lives but now it's become a mechanical chore. When the time for my period approaches I wait with anticipation and dread. We are good people. Our home is full of love. I feel we would make wonderful parents, but it just doesn't seem to happen."

I hear this call for help almost daily. The person speaking and the words change a bit, but each time the feelings are just as desperate. These are the feelings of a couple who is unsuccessfully trying to have a child. Though not always discussed openly and freely, infertility is more common than one might imagine. Our country is filled with people who are concerned with overpopulation and who spend money preventing or terminating unwanted pregnancies. For them, having children is so easy that one need scarcely think about it. Few realize that 15% of couples trying to have a child are unable to do so and that this percentage may rise. When stories are told at social gatherings we may hear about couples who have had immediate success achieving pregnancy. People tend not to speak of what they feel to be their failures. It is very likely that in any group of ten couples of reproductive age at least one person in the room has a reproductive problem or personally knows someone with such a difficulty.

One out of six married couples seek the aid of a physician because of infertility. Following infertility evaluation, the cause of the problem can be determined in about 90% of cases. Nearly 60% of treated couples conceive and this percentage is increasing.

Unlike many other medical problems, infertility is a problem of couples, not individuals. Both members are affected even though only one member may have a physical problem. As a result, infertility tests the very fiber of intimate human relationships.

We have been taught myths and half-truths about producing a pregnancy and occasionally the apparent problems that a couple might experience are based on these errors and nothing more. The purpose of this book is to dispel some of these myths, to explain the process of normal human reproduction, where it may go wrong and what can be done about it.

Great strides have been made in the diagnosis

and treatment of infertility in the last few years and this is just the beginning. There is more hope today than ever before.

We are about to start on the long road of investigation and treatment which hopefully will have at its end the birth of a normal, healthy baby. It is frequently a difficult trip because it is drawn out over several weeks or months and different tests must be timed at various times of the woman's menstrual cycle. Sometimes the test results, instead of answering questions, pose more questions and further studies are required. After a diagnosis is reached and therapy is begun, the more time must pass to see if treatment is successful. Since ovulation usually occurs only once a month, many months may pass before results are seen. This often means that the time necessary to achieve a pregnancy while under therapy for infertility becomes difficult to bear. There are many things couples should know to help sustain them through the evaluation and treatment period. But it is a rare patient who manages to ask all his or her questions, or who can absorb all the information offered by the physician. Often this is a result of the stress of being in a doctor's office.

This book is an attempt to offer what I feel to be the essential information needed by infertility patients to deal with their problems. By understanding why and how tests are done and how these tests really feel, they are easier to tolerate. By understanding why tests are scheduled when they are in relation to the woman's menstrual cycle, the delays in completing the investigation are understood and are less frustrating. By learning how different modes of therapy work, the fact that a couple may not achieve pregnancy immediately is no longer surprising and therefore may be less depressing. It is only by possessing all the information that one can deal with the road traveled to achieve pregnancy with greater ease.

This book is written in "layers" so that it is possible to get a brief discussion of a topic by reading the opening paragraphs, or to get a more extensive explanation of a topic by reading further. Basic ideas and important concepts are repeated from chapter to chapter for emphasis and to facilitate understanding. This repetition also reduces the necessity of turning back and forth from chapter to chapter. An outline presented in the margins will help point out the relationship of ideas and will offer a space for your own notes and thoughts. Illustrations and charts are used extensively to expand and support the discussions.

Specialists in infertility include people of every description, women as well as men. For the sake of editorial consistency, and that alone, I have used the pronoun "he" in the text when referring to the physician.

Let us now take the first step in our journey.

Chapter 1

A Matter of Terms

BEFORE DISCUSSING anything in detail, it is always important to understand the vocabulary that is to be used. Infertility is certainly no exception. The purpose of this chapter is to lay the groundwork for the discussions to follow in the next several chapters. This will be done by presenting the most important terms, defining and then discussing them. Following this, male and female anatomy will be presented and its relevance to infertility briefly reviewed.

I
DEFINITIONS
Infertility

Infertility is the inability of a heterosexual couple to produce a pregnancy after one year of regular intercourse. For a short sentence this definition has a fair number of qualifications in it. It does not simply say, that infertility is the inability for two people to have children. It sets a limit on the amount of time that a couple must try and implies a certain frequency of sexual intercourse. Approximately 80% of sexually active couples of reproductive age will conceive within one year. If an infertility evaluation is begun before this period has passed, then many couples with no reproductive problem will have been studied unnecessarily. In order to achieve a pregnancy a certain number of tries must be made within one year so that there is a sufficient chance of fertilization occurring. Making love every other month for a year would allow insufficient sexual exposure and an inadequate trial to say that infertility exists. It is usually said that a couple should have intercourse approximately every other day around the time of ovulation or every other day throughout the cycle, every month for twelve months without achieving a pregnancy before an infertility evaluation should be considered.

Another use of the word "infertility," refers to the inability of the woman to carry a pregnancy to the point in which it results in the delivery of a live birth. A pregnancy ending in the loss of a fetus before it is able to survive on its own is referred to as a *miscarriage* or an *abortion*. Note that the medical **Miscarriage/** use of the word "abortion" simply means the loss of **Abortion** a fetus before it can survive. It does not imply that the pregnancy has been ended by the administration of any medication or any surgical manipulation. Abortions may further be described as being *spontaneous*, that is, occurring without any Spontaneous manipulation or administration of medication; or it may be referred to as *induced*, implying that Induced something has been done to cause the loss of the pregnancy. *Habitual abortion* refers to spon- Habitual taneous loss of three consecutive pregnancies. The importance of three consecutive losses is significant. There is approximately a 15–20% chance that a woman may lose any pregnancy, without any apparent problem existing. These women usually go on to have uneventful pregnancies and deliveries in the future. Just as there is a certain probability of a woman losing a single pregnancy, there is a certain random chance

15

that two of these fetal losses may occur one after the other. But if three pregnancies are lost in consecutive fashion, then there is a very real possibility of there being something wrong to cause the losses of these pregnancies. A woman who has miscarried once or twice need not necessarily be evaluated for a problem. However, with the loss of three pregnancies there is appropriate indication and justification for medical evaluation. (See Chapter 7.)

The inability to conceive may occur after having another child or may occur without ever having established a pregnancy first. These two possibilities are described by different terms. *Primary infertility* is infertility without any pre-existing pregnancies. *Secondary infertility* is infertility following one or more pregnancies. In the case of secondary infertility, the couple has already demonstrated the ability to produce a child on at least one occasion. In a certain sense they have demonstrated that the basic apparatus is present and capable of working at least once. In primary infertility, the couple has never produced a child. The basic reproductive apparatus has never been shown to work at all. Statistically, primary and secondary infertility each have different causes, though generally the same problems must be considered in each case.

Infertility is a symptom and not a specific disease. It is a manifestation of a problem that exists within a couple. The problem may be within the male or the female, or both. Infertility is unique in that regardless of which individual may have the problem leading to infertility, the couple, rather than the individual is affected.

Approximately 15% or more of couples of

Primary Infertility

Secondary Infertility

reproductive age in the United States are infertile. Of those couples that are infertile, approximately 40% have infertility of male origin and 50% from problems occurring in the female. Previous estimates had been that the remaining 10% had infertility of undetermined cause. This latter category refers to couples who have had a complete infertility evaluation carried out and no reason for infertility could be determined. It does not mean that these patients did not have a problem. It was rather that the specialty of Reproductive Medicine was unable to determine what their problem was. In order to adequately treat a couple, the cause of their infertility must be found. If one is unable to determine the cause, appropriate therapy cannot be instituted. Thus, that group with unexplained infertility represents a particular area of frustration for both patient and physician. With the advances of Reproductive Medicine, that percentage of patients with unexplained infertility has gradually decreased and a recent estimate at this writing has made the group approximately 3.5% rather than 10%. This means that as the science of Reproductive Medicine gradually evolves, we are finding more patients with diagnosable problems and less patients with "unexplained infertility." As more patients have problems that can be diagnosed we have more patients who can be successfully treated. The result is more pregnancies for those patients who desire them.

In order to understand how pregnancy occurs normally, and therefore how it can fail to occur in an infertile couple, one first needs to know a bit of the anatomy of both the normal male and female.

Let us begin with the anatomy of the man. The

**II
ANATOMY
Male**

17

Male reproductive organs

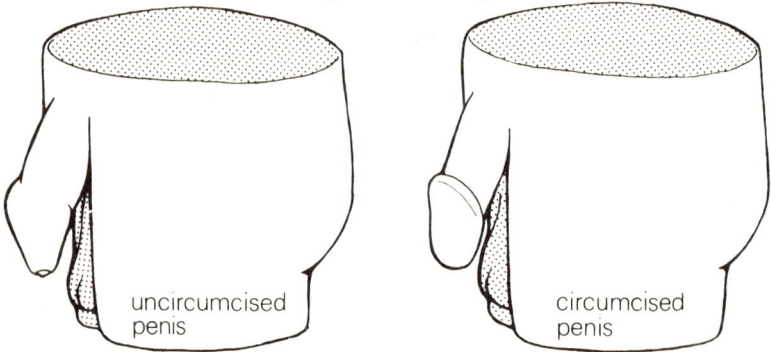

Figure 1.1a *External genitalia*

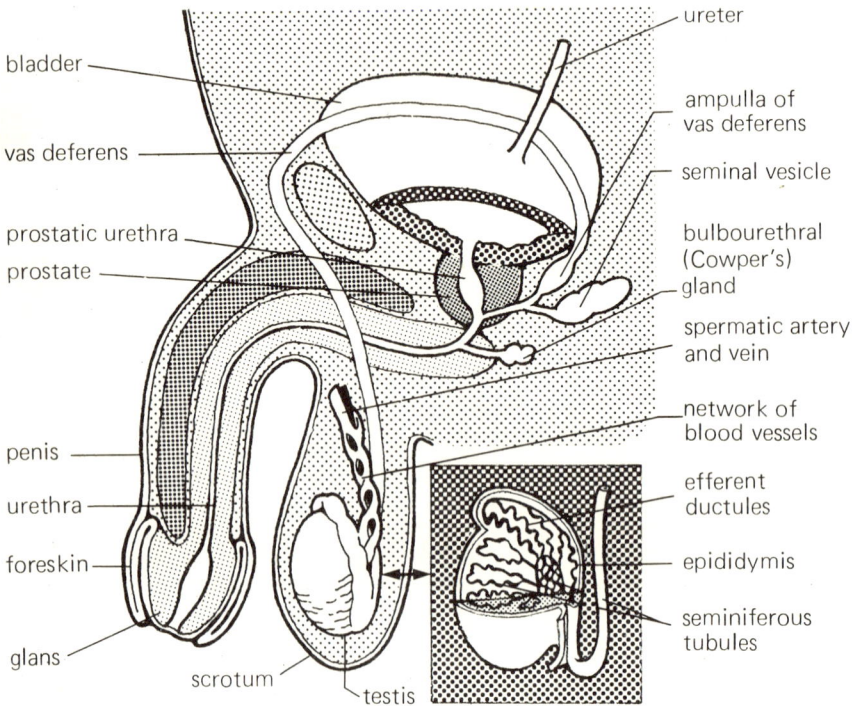

Figure 1.1b *Internal genitalia (cross-section schematic view)*

18

male sex organs consist of a *penis* and *two testes*, sometimes referred to as *testicles*, enclosed within a pouch of skin and fibrous tissue, called the *scrotum*. The *testes* are a source of sperm cells and hormones, most notably *testosterone*. Testosterone is a chemical substance responsible for the shape and characteristics of the male body, such as the texture of skin, hair distribution, voice quality, etc. The testes are connected to the penis by a system of tubes. The testis itself is composed of multiple lobules, each one containing the *seminiferous tubules*, the apparatus necessary to produce many sperm cells. The lobules are connected to small channels which all empty into larger ducts, and finally a structure called the *epididymis*. The epididymis is a somewhat coiled, tubular structure which then directly joins the *vas deferens* which is a somewhat straight, tubular structure. The vas deferens from each testis goes up in the scrotum and enters the penis within the abdomen. The penis has a channel within it called the *urethra*. It is through the urethra that sperm is released and that urine is excreted. The vas deferens joins the urethra by passing through the *ejaculatory ducts* and the *prostate gland.* Sperm is produced within the seminiferous tubules of the testis by a process known as *spermatogenesis*. The sperm enters the network of tubules and eventually gains access to the epididymis. It is within this chamber-like area that further maturation and development of the sperm cells takes place. Within the epididymis sperm cells are moved along by a series of muscular contractions of the tube known as *peristalsis*. From the epididymis the sperm enters the vas deferens and travels up to the area of the prostate. At the point of junction of the vas deferens and the urethra, a small, convoluted, sac-like area called the *seminal vesicle* is found. The sperm produced and carried up through the vas deferens is stored near the seminal vesicle. The stored sperm then enters the urethra where secretions from the seminal vesicle and the prostate are added. The sperm and secretions travel along the urethra and leave the body through the tip of the penis (Figures 1.1a and 1.1b).

Ejaculation, release of sperm at the time of orgasm, occurs when the seminal fluid reaches the area of the urethra that is within the prostate. The fluid and sperm cells are propelled forward by the contractions of the muscles within the penis. The tip of the penis is extensively innervated by sensory nerve endings, and is very sensitive to touch and other forms of stimulation. Its sensitivity and behavior are very much like that of the female clitoris. Upon stimulation, a number of nerve pathways are activated and a muscular ring around the opening of the bladder is caused to close thereby preventing the sperm from entering the bladder. Such a backward release of sperm into the bladder rather than being emitted through the penis is called *retrograde ejaculation.*

The administration of certain drugs such as antidepressants and anti-high blood pressure medications, may diminish the contractile ability of the muscular ring around the opening of the bladder and thereby allow retrograde ejaculation to occur. If this sperm goes backward into the bladder, a very small number of sperm cells may be released through the penis and infertility may result.

The first part of the ejaculate emitted from the penis is rich in sperm while the last part is fluid and contains few sperm cells. If the male has a very low sperm count and a high semen volume it is possible to artificially raise the concentration of his ejaculate by discarding the second sperm poor portion and using only the first, highly concentrated portion for the purpose of producing a pregnancy.

Now that male structure has been reviewed, the next topic is female anatomy. A woman's reproductive organs can arbitrarily be divided into two areas (Figures 1.2a and 1.2b), her external organs or her external genitalia and her internal organs or her internal genitalia.

Female

The *external genitalia* consists of a double set of lip-like structures surrounding the vagina. The inner lips on either side of the vagina are called the *labia minora*. Outside the labia minora are larger lip-like structures called the *labia majora*. The labia minora connect above the vagina and cover a small, highly sensitive erectile structure called the *clitoris*.

External Genitalia

The clitoris is well innervated by many sensory nerve endings and is exquisitely sensitive to touch and stimulation. Part of its response to such stimulation is enlargement and the increase of secretions within the vagina. The clitoris, upon stimulation becomes filled with blood and becomes somewhat erect. It is at this time that it appears very much like a miniature penis in general configuration. Indeed, embryologically, it derives from the same area in the fetus as does the tip of the penis. Just below the clitoris is a small opening called the *urethral meatus* through which a woman urinates. Below this opening is the *vaginal canal*.

The *internal genitalia* are composed of the *vagina*, *cervix*, *uterus*, *Fallopian tubes* and *ovaries*. The *vagina* is a long, tube-like structure, connecting

Internal Genitalia

21

Female reproductive organs

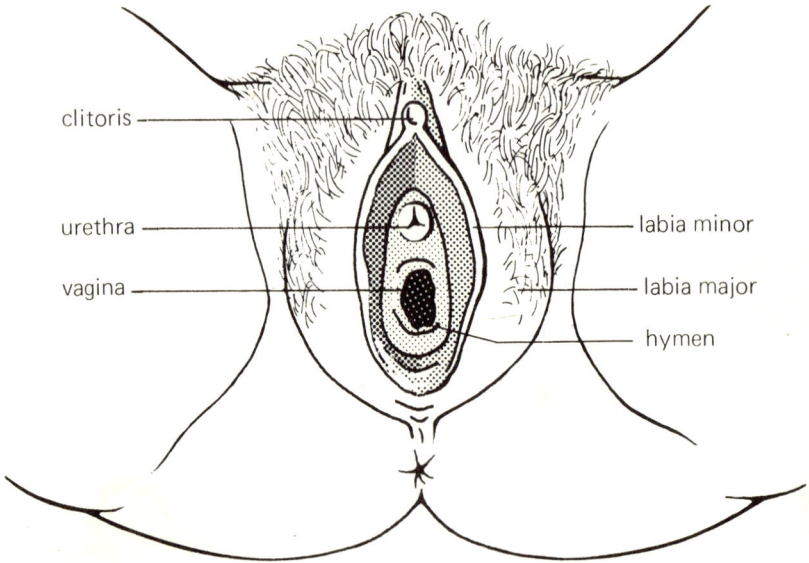

clitoris

urethra

vagina

labia minor

labia major

hymen

Figure 1.2a *External genitalia*

the uterus with the outer world, by way of the external genitalia. At the junction of the vagina with the external genitalia there is a membrane of varying thickness referred to as the *hymen*. After this has been penetrated or broken, the remnants of the hymen remain as small, irregular structures on the side of the vagina. If the hymen is of unusual thickness, penetration of this membrane with a penis or other means, may be impossible. In order to achieve entrance into the vagina in this case, the hymen must be opened surgically. The lining of the vagina is moist membrane constantly producing mucoid secretion. This mucoid fluid maintains the soft, slippery texture of the tissue.

The vagina joins the *womb* or *uterus* at a

22

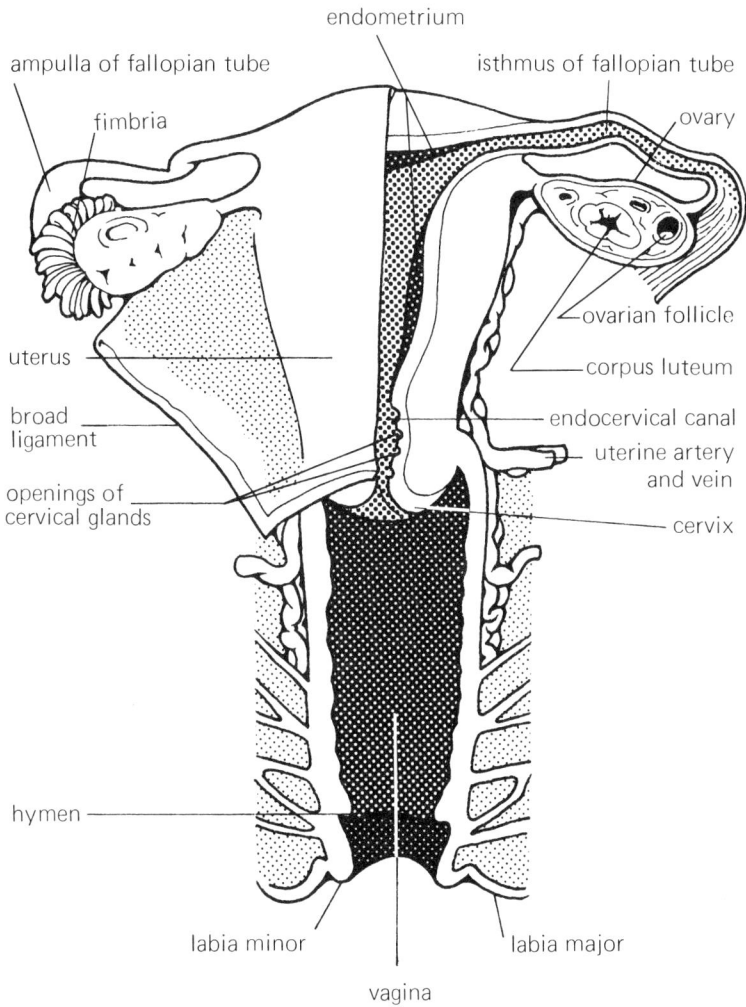

endometrium

ampulla of fallopian tube

isthmus of fallopian tube

fimbria

ovary

ovarian follicle

uterus

corpus luteum

broad ligament

endocervical canal

uterine artery and vein

openings of cervical glands

cervix

hymen

labia minor

labia major

vagina

Figure 1.2b *Internal genitalia (schematic view)*

small, circular area which is called the *cervix*. The uterus is shaped very much like a very thick walled, muscular inverted sack. The opening of the "sack" is the cervix. It is through the cervix that menstrual blood flows out into the vagina. It is also through this opening that sperm enters the uterus on its way into the Fallopian tubes. The uterus has a specialized lining called *endometrium*. This tissue responds to hormonal production by the ovary. At times the uterine lining, the endometrium, grows quite thick. At other times it crumbles and pours out through the cervix into the vagina. When the latter occurs it is known as the woman's *period*, *menses* or *menstrual flow*. The cervix itself is lined by glands which produce mucus. The quality and volume of mucus changes with the woman's cycle. Discussion of the cycle will occur in the next chapter. However, let it suffice for the time being to say that at most times a small amount of very thick mucus is present. At the time of ovulation however, a large amount of very watery mucus is produced by the cervix. This change in the quality of the cervical mucus produces a very favorable medium through which sperm can enter the uterus. When the cervical mucus is very thick and present in small quantities it acts as a barrier, preventing sperm from easily entering the uterus. But when the volume of the cervical mucus is increased and its texture has become watery, sperm can swim through this substance rather than becoming trapped in it. The result is that the cervical mucus favors sperm entering the uterus at the time of ovulation.

The uterus is positioned within the female pelvis. It is most frequently tilted forward, bending toward the front of the woman's abdomen. This uterus is described as being *anteverted* and *anteflexed*. The uterus may rather be tilted backward so that it is bending in the direction of the woman's back. In this case the uterus is described as being *retroverted* and *retroflexed*. The common term for this last situation is a *tipped uterus*. A uterus which is tilted forward is more common that a uterus which is tilted backward. Because something is less common does not mean that it is abnormal. If most people had brown eyes and one person had blue eyes, saying that you have blue eyes does not mean that you have anything wrong with you. It is simply a way of describing a person. Telling a woman that she has a tipped uterus is simply a way of describing the position of the uterus but by itself does not imply that there is anything wrong with the uterus. Approximately 80% of women have an anteverted uterus and 20% have a retroverted uterus (Figures 1.3 and 1.4).

Projecting off each side of the body of the uterus are two tubes. These structures, called the *Fallopian tubes* or *oviducts*, form the passages through which the egg is conducted from the ovary into the uterus. The Fallopian tubes are relatively long structures with specialized funnel-shaped, mobile areas at their outer ends. The funnel-shaped area is called the *fimbria* and is specially designed to pick up eggs. The Fallopian tube itself is a muscular, highly movable tubular structure capable of highly coordinated movement. The lining of the tube is folded and lined with microscopic hair-like projections called *cilia*, each capable of creating highly coordinated movements. The tubal lining, called the *endosalpinx*, is also capable of producing a fluid that can act as a nutritive medium for the egg. The

25

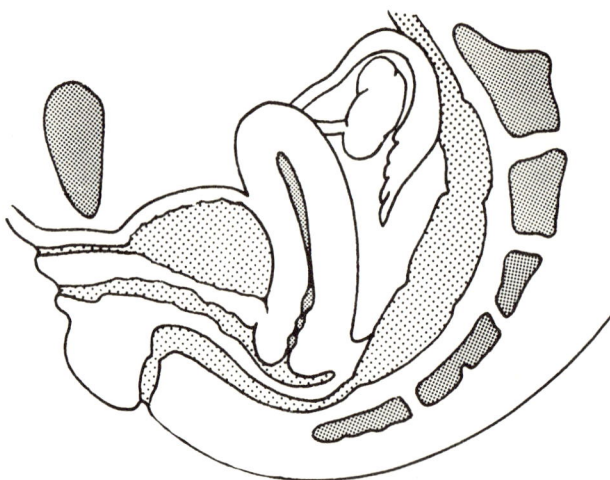

Figure 1.3 *An anteverted or normally positioned uterus*

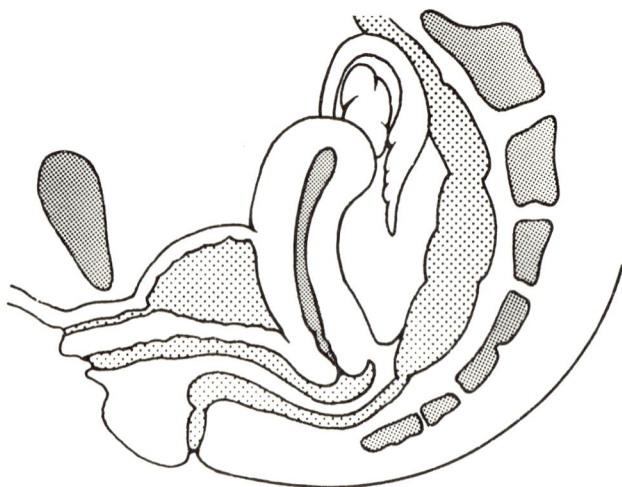

Figure 1.4 *Retroverted or tipped uterus*

fertilized egg is conducted down the oviduct by the contractions of its muscular wall and by the beating of the cilia.

The *ovaries* are ovoid-shaped structures the size and shape of an olive. They are found just under the Fallopian tubes, and to the side of the body of the uterus. The ovaries release an *ovum* (egg) at the time of ovulation. Ovaries are also the source of hormones such as *estrogen* and *progesterone*. At the time of ovulation the ovary releases an egg which is picked up by the fimbria. The ovum is conducted through the internal channel of the Fallopian tube to approximately the middle third of the tube. If the male and female make love at the time of ovulation, the sperm will mix with the watery cervical mucus and swim through the cervix into the uterine cavity. The sperm will be actively conducted through the uterine cavity into the Fallopian tubes. A sperm cell and the ovum which was released will unite by a process called *fertilization*. The fertilized ovum then moves through the Fallopian tube into the uterine cavity where it attaches to the uterine lining. This newly fertilized egg grows into an embryo, a fetus, and later, a baby.

The meanings of the terms "primary" and "secondary" infertility and "habitual abortion" have been reviewed. The anatomy of the reproductive organs of both the male and the female have been discussed. The next problem that must be reviewed is at what point should a couple decide that they have an infertility problem. At what point should a couple seek the advice of a physician for the problems of infertility? The definition of infertility specifies that a couple should have regular sexual relations for at least one year without con-

**III
WHEN SHOULD
A COUPLE BE
EVALUATED?**

Infertility

ception. As mentioned earlier, regular sexual relations is taken to mean making love every other day around ovulation time, or every other day throughout the cycle, every month for twelve months. At this point in our discussion it may not be obvious as to how the determination of ovulation time is made. This will be discussed at length in a later chapter. This "one year period" applies whether or not the couple has previously achieved pregnancy.

Miscarriage

If, on the other hand, the couple has achieved pregnancy and three consecutive pregnancies have ended spontaneously without the birth of a live child, then that too is an indication for seeking medical help. As with anything, these are only guidelines, they are not absolute rules. They are set up so that those people who have the greatest need may get attention while those couples who have the greatest probability of having no problem will not be made to begin an unnecessary infertility investigation. Approximately 80% of those patients who have had a single miscarriage will go on to have families with no problems. On the other hand, approximately 80% of those patients who have had three or more spontaneous abortions, (miscarriages), will be found to have some cause for their problem. Eighty percent of those patients who attempt pregnancy will conceive within one year of regular sexual activity. With these statistics it will be apparent that only those patients who have had three or more miscarriages or who have been trying to achieve a pregnancy for a year or more would best be served by beginning an infertility evaluation.

As said earlier, these are not absolute rules and must be tempered by the judgment of the physician.

It is apparent that if on initial review of the history, the man is unable to ejaculate, i.e., release semen from his penis on orgasm, or that it is unlikely that the woman is ovulating at all, there would be nothing gained by waiting a full year before beginning evaluation.

The evaluation is often feared to be painful, very long in duration and extremely costly. This is usually not the case. The period of time for evaluation depends upon the kinds of problems the studies find. Usually, the time frame is of the order of several weeks to months. The cost varies tremendously but if finances are a problem, infertility clinics usually are available in most areas. Discomfort is a very private matter. What is tolerable to one person may be agony to another. Nevertheless, it is my experience that in the hands of an experienced practitioner, the infertility workup can take place with a minimal degree of discomfort. I do not say this as a disinterested third party, but as a human being strongly involved in the feelings of my patients. I could not bring myself to cause repeated or significant discomfort to anyone if this appeared to be the case.

IV EVALUATION: COST AND DISCOMFORT

Now that the basics have been presented, the next step is to see how everything fits together for the production of a pregnancy. The next chapter will discuss this in detail.

Chapter 2

Baby Production:
the way it should work

AT FIRST IT APPEARS that producing a child is really not terribly difficult. All that is required is that one healthy sperm and a healthy egg, an *ovum*, be in the same place at the same time so that the two can unite. The resulting fertilized ovum then must be kept in a protected area for approximately forty weeks and given proper nourishment and room to grow. Any interruption in this basic scheme preventing the egg and sperm from uniting or making it impossible for the fertilized egg to develop, will result in infertility. The ways this scheme can be interrupted are many. Before one can understand what can go wrong, one must first understand what happens when things work properly. That is the purpose of this chapter.

I
BASIC SCHEME

After a normal menstrual flow, several eggs within the woman's ovary begin to develop. Soon, one of these developing eggs matures more than the rest and in approximately fourteen days after the onset of the woman's menstrual flow, this mature egg pops out of the surface of the ovary. This is known as *ovulation*. A specialized, funnel-shaped structure at the end of the Fallopian tube called the *fimbria* will pick up this egg and the lining of the

Ovulation

Egg Picked Up

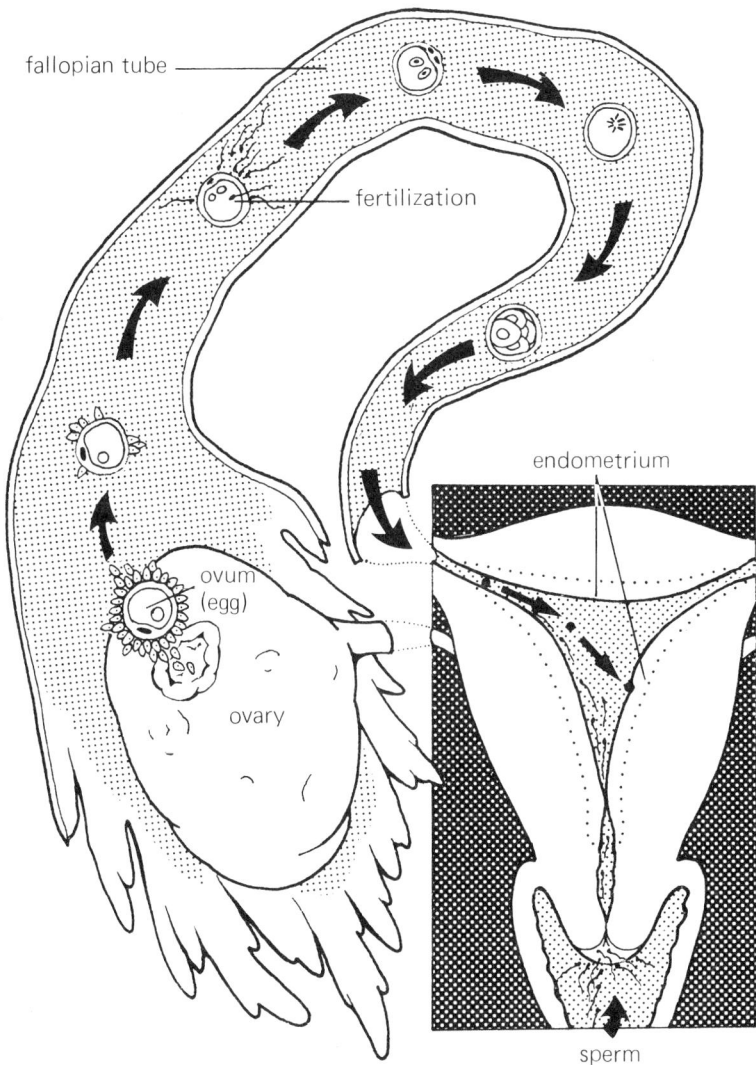

Figure 2.1 *Ovulation and fertilization*

Sperm

Fertilization

Implantation

**II
DETAILED
SCHEME**

tube will move the egg down the oviduct to approximately the middle third of the tube. If a couple has sexual relations at this time, sperm released by the penis is placed within the vagina next to the *cervix*, (the opening of the womb). The sperm cells swim through the cervical mucus at the opening of the uterus (the womb), and are carried into the cavity of the uterus and up into the Fallopian tube. This trip takes only about ten to twenty minutes. The sperm and the egg are now in the same place and by random movement, hopefully, one sperm cell will meet this egg and the two will unite causing *fertilization*. The fertilized egg now begins to move down the tube again, toward the uterus. It crosses into the uterine cavity, the space within the uterus, and adheres to the lining of this cavity. This is called *implantation*. The tissue lining the wall is very thick, filled with blood vessels, and capable of delivering nourishment to this newly fertilized ovum. The fertilized egg quickly develops and progresses into an embryo, eventually a fetus, and then a new human being. As time passes, the *placenta*, a specialized organ within the uterine cavity connecting the fetus to the mother, will grow providing nutrition and respiration to this developing fetus.

This discussion started by simply saying that ovulation (the release of an egg) occurred, but ovulation does not just happen without preparation. Eggs do not just develop in the ovary, mature and pop out of the surface without an appropriate stimulus. Furthermore, the lining of the uterus has to be carefully prepared so that the fertilized ovum can implant onto it. The body requires some kind of mechanism to control the release of the egg and the development of the lining of the uterus in a synchronous manner. This is necessary so that when the egg finally gets to the uterine cavity, the lining is prepared to support it for many weeks in its development toward becoming a human being. This is how it happens.

In the floor of the brain is a gland called the *pituitary gland*. This is sometimes called the "master gland" because it controls the functioning of many other glands distributed throughout the body. Just above the pituitary is a section of the brain called the *hypothalamus* which in turn controls the pituitary gland and is itself controlled by higher centers of the brain. The result is a neurological system in which components are interconnected like the wires of a vast telephone network. Though the pituitary gland produces many hormones, at this moment we are interested only in two, one called *FSH*, follicle stimulating hormone, and the other, *LH*, luteinizing hormone. FSH and LH are released into the bloodstream and when they reach the ovary they stimulate the ovary so that estrogen is produced and several eggs begin to ripen. The estrogen produced by the ovary enters the blood and is distributed throughout the body. It is *estrogen* that is important in determining the shape of the female's body, the development of her breasts, the texture of her skin, the development and texture of her hair and even the secretions within her vagina. Estrogen also stimulates the lining of the uterus to grow in a very specific manner, (i.e., to proliferate and grow thicker). The sexually mature woman seems to have a clock-like mechanism within the hypothalamus that is called the *cyclic center*. At a certain time in the woman's cycle the

Pituitary Gland

Hypothalamus

Pituitary Hormones
FSH
LH

Ovary
Estrogen

Cyclic Center of Hypothalamus

33

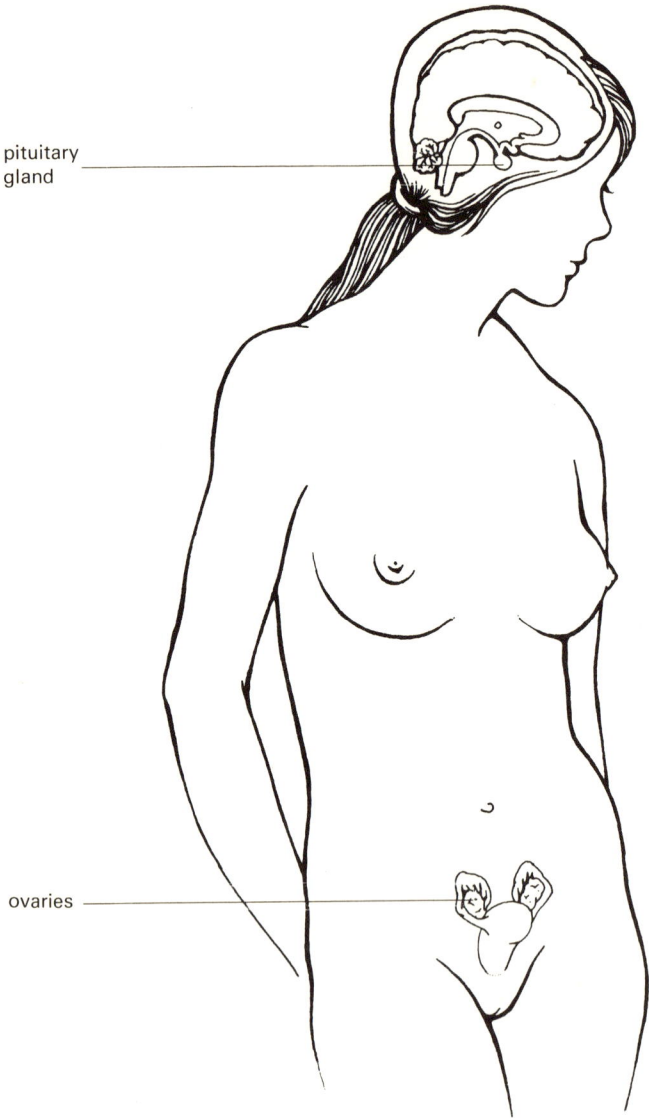

pituitary
gland

ovaries

Figure 2.2 *The location of the pituitary gland and the ovaries*

cyclic center of the hypothalamus triggers the release of a large amount of FSH and LH from the pituitary gland and causes that developing ovum which is most mature to be released by the ovary, thus causing ovulation. (See Figures 2.2, 2.3a, 2.3b.)

After ovulation, the area of the ovary from which the egg was released is converted to a very specialized structure called a *corpus luteum.* These **Corpus Luteum** words mean the "yellow body" and if one looks at the surface of the ovary, one sees exactly what the words suggest, a localized, yellow structure. The corpus luteum produces another hormone called progesterone. *Progesterone* enters the circulatory Progesterone system and, when it reaches the tissue lining the uterus, it causes a change in the structure of the lining, so that it can better provide support and nourishment to the newly fertilized egg. It takes approximately five days for the newly fertilized egg to reach the lining of the uterus. This insures enough time for the uterine lining to develop the appropriate tissue which can best keep this developing human being alive. (See Figure 2.3c.)

And so the same mechanisms that allow for the development of an egg and its release from the surface of the ovary also allow for the preparation of the lining of the uterus to properly accept and maintain the fertilized egg.

The corpus luteum, the "yellow body," may be thought of as a factory within the surface of the ovary producing progesterone. This progesterone factory is controlled by the pituitary gland and, if pregnancy does not occur, the factory fails and shuts off after fourteen days of functioning. Thus, progesterone production stops and the uterine lining

Interaction of the pituitary and the ovary (Schematic)

Figure 2.3a

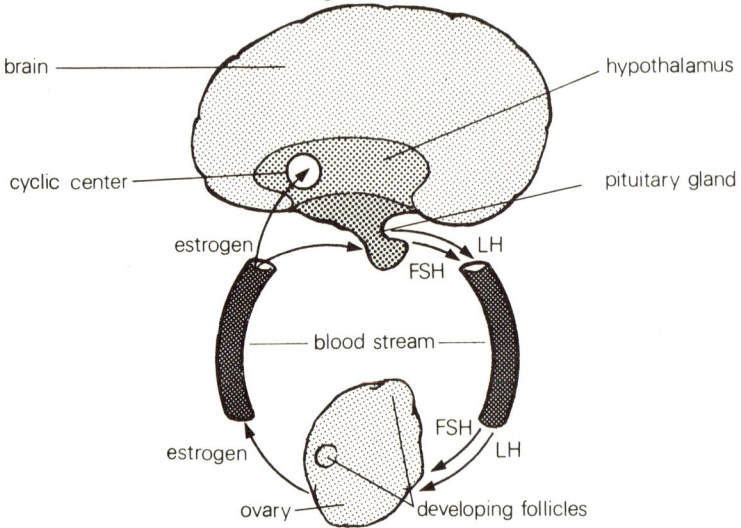

can no longer be maintained in its preparatory state. With the cessation of progesterone production the uterine lining crumbles and sloughs. The entire lining is shed over a three to five day interval and when it flows out through the cervix and into the vagina it is recognized as the woman's menstrual period.

If pregnancy is to occur, the lining of the uterus must be maintained by progesterone for longer than the fourteen day usual life of the corpus luteum. Thus, if an egg is fertilized and pregnancy does occur, the newly developing placental tissue takes control of the corpus luteum and keeps it functioning into the early weeks of pregnancy.

Menstrual Cycle   The normal woman releases an egg from her ovary about once a month. As discussed, if she does

Figure 2.3b   **Figure 2.3c**

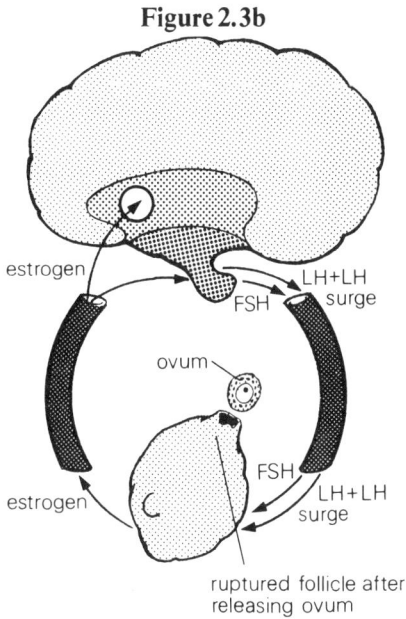

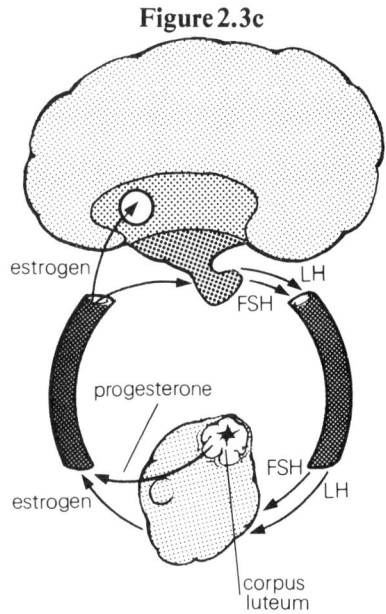

Figure 2.3a *The pituitary produces FSH and LH which enter the bloodstream. These hormones act on the ovary causing some follicles to ripen and estrogen to be produced. Estrogen then enters the bloodstream and acts on the hypothalamus and pituitary, modifying the amount of FSH and LH produced. In this way a completely interacting circuit is established.*

Figure 2.3b *In order for ovulation to occur, a sudden massive amount of LH must be released from the pituitary. When this happens a ripened follicle bursts and an ovum (egg) is released from the surface of the ovary. This massive release of LH producing ovulation is called the LH surge.*

Figure 2.3c *After ovulation, the corpus luteum, found in the site of the ruptured follicle, produces progesterone.*

not become pregnant she will get her menstrual flow fourteen days after ovulation. The interval of time from the first day of bleeding in one month to the first day of bleeding in the next month is referred to

as the menstrual cycle. The days of the menstrual cycle are numbered consecutively from the first day of vaginal bleeding. The first day of the menstrual flow is always called cycle day one regardless of what the calendar date might be. Lois's period began on August 20 and so, for her, August 20 was cycle day one of that menstrual cycle.

The most common length of a menstrual cycle is twenty-eight days with ovulation occurring on cycle day fourteen. Estrogen is produced by the ovary during the entire menstrual cycle but progesterone is produced only from ovulation to just before the onset of menses, (cycle day fourteen to twenty-eight).

Uterine Lining
Proliferative
Endometrium
(Estrogen)

When estrogen acts alone on the uterine lining it produces a characteristic tissue called *proliferative endometrium*. After ovulation, when progesterone is produced by the corpus luteum in addition to the estrogen, the uterine lining is converted to

Secretory
Endometrium
(Progesterone)

secretory endometrium. It is secretory endometrium that is prepared to receive and nourish the newly fertilized ovum. The secretory endometrium changes in structure each day under the influence of progesterone. The changes are so precise and predictable that it is possible to look at the microscopic structure of a piece of secretory endometrium and to know how many days earlier ovulation occurred. (See Figure 2.4.)

Parts of Cycle

For the sake of further discussion, the first half of the menstrual cycle when estrogen alone is being

Proliferative Phase produced, is called the *proliferative phase* of the

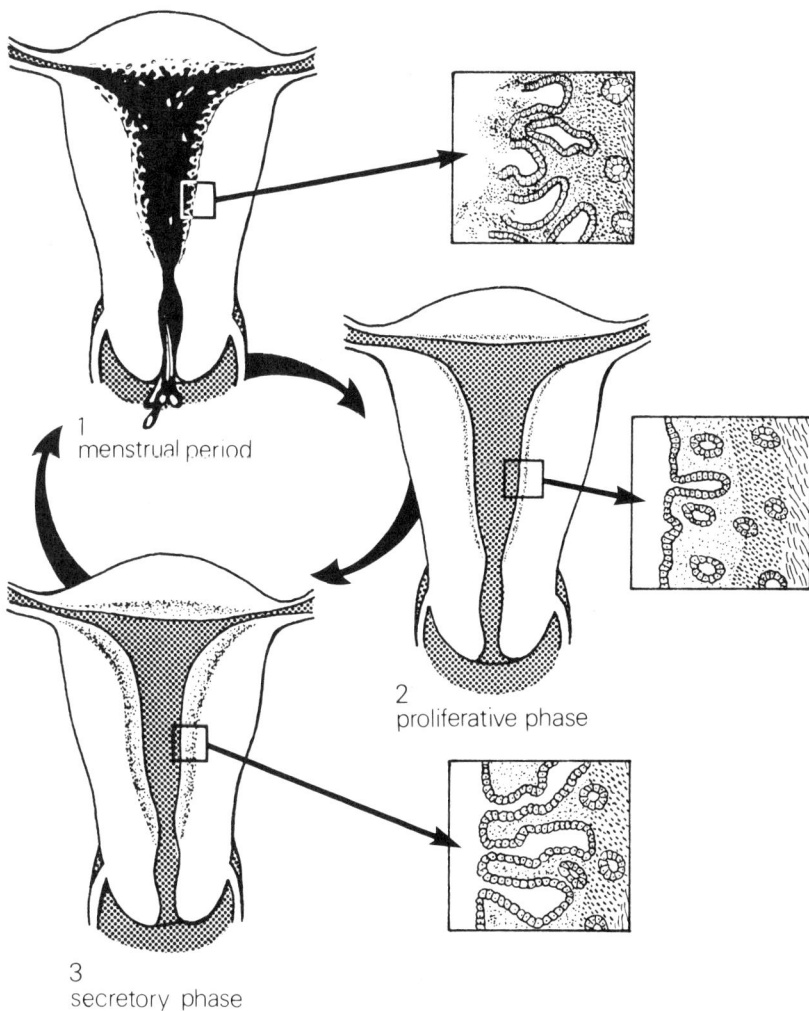

1
menstrual period

2
proliferative phase

3
secretory phase

Figure 2.4 *Phases of the menstrual cycle. The lining of the uterus grows and changes during the menstrual cycle. During the* proliferative phase *it grows and thickens. In the* secretory phase *it is readied to receive a fertilized egg. If pregnancy does not occur, the lining crumbles and is seen as the woman's menstrual flow.*

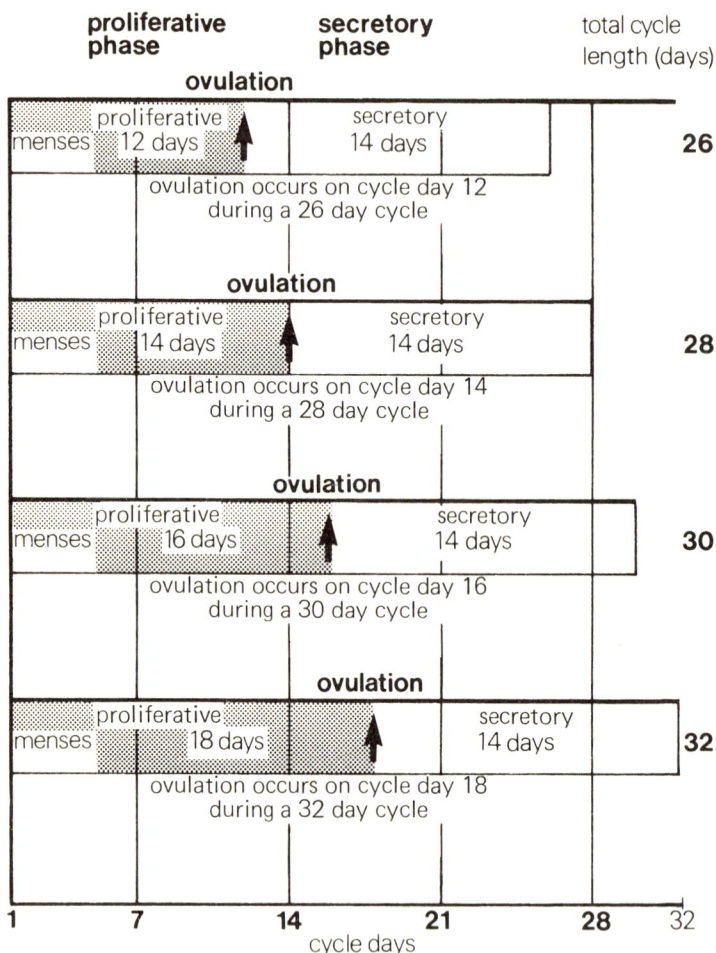

Figure 2.5 *Numbering the days of the menstrual cycle.
The first day of a woman's menstrual period (menses) is called
cycle day one. The second half of the menstrual cycle, the
secretory phase, is fixed at fourteen days in length, while the
first half, the proliferative phase, varies with the length of the
cycle. Ovulation occurs at the end of the proliferative phase.
By subtracting fourteen from the total number of days of
the menstrual cycle, one gets the day of theoretical ovulation.*

cycle. Similarly, the second half of the cycle is called the *secretory phase*. The second half, or secretory phase, is fixed at fourteen days, but the first half, or proliferative phase, can vary in length from woman to woman, or even in the same woman, from cycle to cycle. If a woman has a twenty-eight day menstrual cycle she has a fourteen day proliferative phase, ovulates on cycle day fourteen and has a fourteen day secretory phase. If her cycle is thirty days in length, the first half of her cycle is sixteen days long with ovulation occurring on cycle day sixteen. Similarly, if the female has a twenty-five day cycle that means that the proliferative phase is eleven days long and that ovulation occurs on cycle day eleven. In women who have cycles of varying lengths, it is always the first half of the cycle that varies in duration while the second half remains fixed. Since ovulation occurs at the end of the proliferative phase and it may vary in length, it may be difficult to determine exactly when ovulation occurs, in a woman with a variable cycle, while that cycle is occurring. However, when menses occur, all the woman has to do to determine when the ovum was released is to count back fourteen days. Unfortunately, this is after the fact and this method is of less than ideal help during the cycles that a couple is attempting pregnancy. (See Figure 2.5.)

Secretory Phase

Fertilization is a random thing. Though that statement sounds like a 1938 song title, it has a great deal of significance. A sperm and an egg may both be in the same area of the tube at the same time. The two meet by random movement, or dumb luck, if you will. As if to increase the chances of fertilization, nature allows not one, but hundreds of thousands of sperm cells to arrive in the tube in the

Fertilization

41

area of the egg. The greater the number of sperm around the egg, the greater the chance of one of those sperm meeting and fertilizing that egg. Still, even if a couple has intercourse on the day before, the day of, and the day after ovulation, pregnancy usually does not occur during the first cycle. It can take up to one year, twelve cycles of regular sexual activity or more, for a normal couple to achieve a pregnancy.

The basic mechanisms of ovulation and fertilization have been presented. In the next chapter some of the errors and myths that are commonly accepted as truth will be discussed.

Chapter 3

Myths, Misconceptions and Misinformation

NOW THAT THE BASIC mechanisms involved in ovulation and the establishment of pregnancy have been reviewed, some of the fables and misinformation regarding human reproduction will be discussed. Based on the information presented so far, some of these statements will seem ridiculous when they are presented. Nevertheless, it is important to explore them to underline their inaccuracy and to emphasize the general concepts presented thus far.

Pregnancy always occurs immediately if intercourse has occurred at ovulation time.
The meeting of the sperm and the egg occurs by random movement. Thus, even though a man and a woman may have intercourse at the right time of the woman's cycle and sperm cells may enter the female reproductive tract, it does not necessarily follow that a sperm and an egg will actually meet. Since fertilization takes place by the random meeting of the sperm and the egg, a number of attempts are necessary for an egg to become fertilized. Given enough tries, over enough cycles, the chances that fertilization will take place are generally good.

Approximately 25% of couples attempting pregnancy will achieve it within one month. Approximately 80% of couples will conceive within one year's time. It is because of this that couples are usually not investigated for infertility unless they have attempted pregnancy with regular sexual relations for twelve cycles and have failed to conceive. Both theory and statistics show that pregnancy usually does not occur right away even if sexual activity was perfectly timed.

In summary — failing to achieve conception after a single cycle is not a sign of a problem.

Ovulation alternates from one ovary one month to the opposite ovary the next month.
Ovulation does not alternate from one ovary to the other. Over the course of the year each ovary appears to ovulate approximately an equal number of times, but the pattern is random rather than alternating. At the beginning of a cycle it is impossible to predict which ovary will be the one to release an egg. Ovulation may occur from the right ovary one month but the following month the chances are just as great that ovulation will occur from the right ovary again as from the left one.

The picture becomes more complicated because it is not always the tube on the same side as the ovary that picks up the egg. It is known that in some rare cases an ovum has been released by one ovary and picked up by the opposite tube. These are women who had only one tube and one ovary each on opposite sides who have achieved pregnancy. What appears to have happened is that the egg was released by the ovary and the tube on the opposite side crossed over to pick it up. These are unusual cases. In the vast majority of women, the tube on the same side picks up the freshly released egg.

Thus, it is not true that ovulation alternates from one ovary to the other. One is unable to predict which ovary will release an egg during any given cycle, and one is even unable to know with certainty which tube will pick up the egg.

Menses indicate ovulation has occurred.
Another way of stating this widely held chestnut is by saying, "If you had a period, you know you have ovulated." Both of these statements are frequently made and both are quite false. Menses indicate only that the lining of the uterus has been partially or completely shed. This usually occurs fourteen days after an ovulation if pregnancy has not occurred. However, if ovulation fails to occur the lining of the uterus may continue to grow as a proliferative endometrium. A proliferative endometrium has very little structural rigidity to it. After several weeks the lining becomes taller and thicker and progressively more brittle. A point is reached where, like piling too many building blocks one on top of the other, the lining outgrows its structural support and begins to crumble. At this time the tissue breaks off and flows out of the cervix into the vagina and appears very much like the menses following an ovulation. In this case however, bleeding that occurs does not follow an ovulation. This is called non-ovulatory or *anovulatory bleeding.*

Anovulatory bleeding, since it is the result of random breaking and sloughing of tissue, may produce almost any kind of menstrual pattern. The woman may experience a menstrual flow that appears to be normal both in amount and duration or she may experience extremely light or extremely heavy vaginal bleeding. Bleeding may go on for several hours or may continue for weeks or months. The point is that vaginal bleeding, menses, does not necessarily mean that ovulation has occurred.

After the age of thirty, you had better not try to get pregnant because the chances of an abnormal child are very, very high.
With increasing age the chances of a woman delivering an abnormal child increases slightly. After the age of thirty-five however, with each increasing year thereafter, the chances of an abnormal newborn increase significantly. Similarly, the chances of a complication occurring to the mother during pregnancy also increases year by year after the age of thirty-five. During the same period of time a woman's spontaneous fertility seems to decrease. This almost seems to be an inborn protective mechanism for the mother, child and species. In summary, fetal and maternal complications increase while spontaneous female fertility decreases after the age of thirty-five. Though this has been supported by numerous studies, recent investigation has questioned these findings. It may be the case that the increase in fetal abnormality and maternal risk may be much less than initially anticipated. Only further studies by other investigators can confirm this.

Recently, it has become possible to obtain information about the unborn baby. While in the uterus, the fetus floats in a water-like environment called the *amniotic fluid.* It sheds cells and body chemicals into this liquid world. By inserting a long hypodermic needle through the abdomen and the uterus into the amniotic fluid, some of this material can be withdrawn and tests performed. The procedure of sampling the amniotic fluid is called *amniocentesis* and is usually done between the fourteenth and sixteenth week of pregnancy. One of the most common and significant tests done is the genetic study which can diagnose certain abnormalities such as *Down's Syndrome*, previously known as Mongolism. (See Figure 3.1.)

By utilizing the information obtained from the amniotic fluid studies it is possible to tell a couple whether or not some of the disorders found in the children of older mothers exist in the unborn child. If such a problem is discovered, the couple may elect to end the pregnancy and thereby prevent the birth of an abnormal child. Using such an approach the risk of a mother above the age of thirty-five having an abnormal child can be sharply reduced.

Based on current information, telling a woman between the ages of thirty to thirty-four not to consider childbearing, as cited above, would be overcautious and unfortunate. However, considering childbearing after the age of thirty-five deserves a significant amount of thought.

If you are frigid you cannot conceive.
Failing to be able to be sexually aroused rarely has a direct effect on being able to become pregnant. If frigidity results in a decreased frequency of sexual relations, then pregnancy becomes more difficult because there is less sexual exposure, rather than resulting from the frigidity itself. If the frigidity is a result of a structural problem within the woman's vagina or certain hormonal deficiencies, then these problems may in turn interfere with fertility. But the

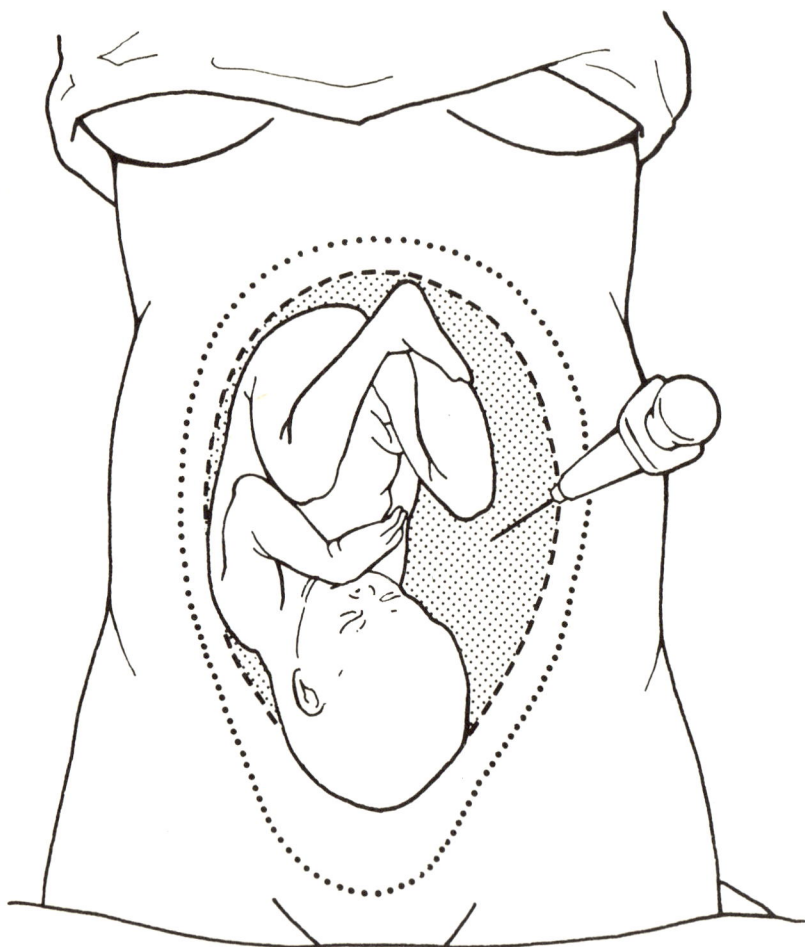

Figure 3.1 *Amniocentesis: the removal of some of the amniotic fluid to evaluate the condition of the fetus.*

failure to be sexually stimulated and aroused in no way prevents ovulation and the ultimate union of a sperm and an egg. Though sexual arousal and satisfaction makes coital activity more satisfying and gratifying, it is not necessary to produce a child.

A "tipped uterus" makes it difficult to become pregnant.
Some twenty years ago this was a widely held belief both among physicians and the interested general public. It was felt that if the uterus was tipped backward it would be more difficult for sperm to enter the uterus and Fallopian tubes and therefore, the chances of conception were diminished. Later studies showed that the incidence of pregnancy among women with retroverted uteri, (wombs that are tipped backward), is approximately the same as women with uteri in the usual position.

Occasionally a woman with a retroverted uterus does have an infertility problem. The womb may be held in the backward position as a result of some pelvic scarring, be it endometriosis or pelvic adhesions (see Chapter 4). In this case, the process that produced the scarring may also have scarred the Fallopian tubes making it difficult for these structures to pick up an egg. Here again, it is not the fact that the uterus is tilted backward that causes the problem but rather the scarring process that may result in infertility. It must be emphasized however, that the vast majority of women with a "tipped womb" have this on a congenital basis (have been born with this), rather than as a result of any pelvic disease. The words "retroverted uterus" or "tipped" or "tilted uterus" should not be taken as meaning that there is anything wrong. It describes something that is uncommon, but it does not mean that there is anything wrong. By itself, a tipped or retroverted uterus is just a variation of normal.

Infertility may be the result of a uterus that is too small.
Like the above, this too was a widely held belief fifteen to twenty years ago. Like many things, old ideas die hard. It used to be felt that the woman with a small uterus was unable to become pregnant simply because the uterus was too small to hold a pregnancy. It has since been shown that with the onset of pregnancy, most of these small uteri previously described as *juvenile*, will easily enlarge to accommodate a growing fetus. Thus, a small uterus by itself is an insufficient reason for infertility.

When a couple has an infertility problem it is best for them to make love with the woman lying on her back with a pillow beneath her buttocks and for the man to assume a position on top of her. Upon completing relations, the woman should raise her legs against a wall and stay in this position for several hours. Another variation of this is: **you are not getting pregnant because you are using the wrong position when making love.**
Unfortunately, there is no magic position that makes pregnancy significantly more likely. If the instructions given above were truly successful, then the best means of *contraception* would be to avoid the position described and for a woman to jump up and down after sex to dislodge the sperm. This particular means of contraception was practiced at the turn of the century but unfortunately, with no demonstrable success.

At the time of ovulation, the cervix is surrounded by a large volume of very watery mucus. This is produced by the cervix and seems to act as an excellent medium to trap sperm cells and to aid them on their trip into the uterine cavity on their way to the Fallopian tube. Once sperm is deposited in the area of the cervix it takes only ten to twenty minutes for it to travel from the cervical mucus up to the Fallopian tube. This seems to be the case regardless of what positions are used during intercourse. Since the basic trip only takes ten to twenty minutes, suggesting that a woman place herself in a position to facilitate sperm movement into her reproductive tract, and to hold that position for several hours, seems illogical and unnecessary. A couple should have intercourse without using lubricants such as petroleum jelly, using whatever techniques they find pleasurable and the woman should linger in bed for approximately thirty minutes after intercourse in any recumbent position she finds comfortable. In this way, ample opportunity is given for the sperm to enter the uterus and Fallopian tubes without the need for utilizing uncomfortable and unnecessary positions.

If you want to get pregnant go on a vacation.
This is a frequently heard suggestion. It is usually followed by a story of a friend, neighbor or relative who had an infertility problem and then finally conceived following a vacation. If infertility is a symptom of an underlying problem influencing the reproductive system then what can a vacation do? How can the stories be explained?

The explanation is fairly simple. Approximately 5% of infertility couples conceive without any therapy. This is the *spontaneous fertility rate* of infertile couples. In order to say that any treatment actually does something for the patient it must be shown to have a higher success rate than 5% – the pregnancy rate when no treatment is done. If a drug or operation is associated with a 5% pregnancy rate then it can be assumed the treatment was of little or no help at all. On the other hand, if couples were given an unrelated therapy such as having rocks taped to their armpits, a certain percentage, the same 5%, will conceive. Vacations fit into this last category. They may be enjoyable in themselves, but as a treatment for infertility they appear to be no more successful than doing nothing at all.

I have heard of infertile couples who adopt a child and then are able to have a child of their own. So, if you are having trouble getting pregnant, first adopt. The pregnancy rate following adoption is the same as the rate when no treatment is given. Thus, adoption can be shown to do nothing to improve the chances of conception. The explanation is the same as just presented for the effect of vacations on infertility.

More importantly, adopting a child is indeed one approach to the treatment of infertility, but not in the way the above misconception suggests. Adoption is an end in itself directly fulfilling the needs of a child and a couple. It must not be thought of as a means of inducing a pregnancy. With the increased use of contraception and the liberal use of abortion, the number of adoptable children is vastly reduced. In my opinion, these children should be considered for couples who, in spite of treatment cannot conceive, and not as therapy to assist conception.

Infertility is usually a result of a problem with the female member of the couple.

This frequently stated observation borders on being a wholesale slander leveled against women. It has resulted in needless grief and guilt, and has actually prevented proper infertility evaluation by making some men unwilling to be studied. The precise numbers that one can present to counter this ridiculous statement may differ depending upon which studies one wishes to refer to. In general, one can say that male problems account for 40% of infertility, female problems account for 50% and in 10% of couples no cause for infertility can be found. Thus, it is about as likely that infertility may be due to the male as to the female partner.

More importantly, such a statement reflects a desire to assign fault to one member of a couple. It is not important who has the medical difficulty because it shows itself as a problem of the couple and not the individual, and must be approached as such. Furthermore, we do not usually feel guilty or make others feel guilty when they have medical problems. No one directs blame at an individual with an ulcer, or gall stones. Infertility is a symptom of a medical dysfunction and should be approached no differently than any other medical problem.

Some of the myths and misconceptions that have surrounded infertility have just been reviewed. I certainly have not covered all of them but it is clear that many widely held views are filled with inaccuracies. Having pointed out the inaccuracies, let us now progress to the next chapter which will discuss the causes of infertility.

Chapter 4

The Causes of Infertility

BEFORE ONE CAN understand how to help a couple achieve a pregnancy one must understand what are the possible reasons for that couple having been unsuccessful up to this point. A previous chapter described ovulation, the pathway the sperm follows in reaching the egg, fertilization and the trip of the fertilized egg back to the protection of the uterus. A problem in any one of these steps, plus several not yet presented, will break the sequence of things and pregnancy will not occur. Since there are many steps in "baby production" and any one or more of them may go wrong resulting in infertility, the surprising thing is that anyone has been able to have a child at all.

For the purposes of this book, the causes of infertility will be grouped into six categories.

I.   Male Factor – a problem in the male sex partner resulting in poor sperm production.

II. Female Factor – a problem in the female sex partner stemming from lack of ovulation, a hormonal imbalance and/or a structural abnormality.

III. Male–Female Interaction.

IV. Psychological Factor.
V. Genetic Factor.
VI. Infertility of Undetermined Cause.

The first major category, *male factor infertility*, is implicated when a microscopic examination of the male's sperm, a *semen analysis*, reveals that the man is producing too few sperm to be able to fertilize a normal woman. It is not the mere number of sperm cells that are produced that is important. The male must also produce an adequate percentage of motile (moving) normally shaped sperm cells, for it is only normally shaped, motile cells that are capable of fertilizing an egg. It is possible for a male to produce a semen specimen with an adequate number of sperm cells but with too few of those cells that are both normal in shape and motility to produce a pregnancy. Abnormalities in the semen specimen indicate the need to evaluate the male sex partner by a urologist specializing in male infertility. Hormonal studies including thyroid and adrenal tests, and physical examination, looking for abnormalities of the testes should be done. (See Figure 4.1.)

I
MALE FACTOR
Semen Analysis

Male infertility problems may be a result of several categories of defects. These general categories are as follows: structural problems, problems related to infection, genetic problems, hormonal problems, drug problems, environmental problems and the general category referred to as "other."

Problems

Structural problems that may result in male infertility are diverse in nature. The *varicocele* is a grossly enlarged series of veins around the epididymis and the vas deferens of the testes. It

Structural
Varicocele

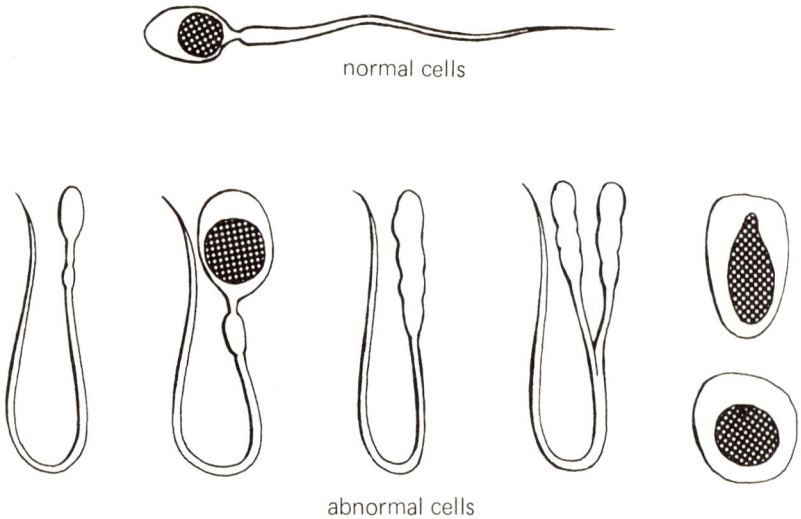

normal cells

abnormal cells

Figure 4.1 *Semen analysis. Not all the sperm cells produced are of normal shape. Both normal and abnormal forms are shown.*

results in infertility by mechanisms that are still being debated at this point. There is no explanation that seems to apply to all cases uniformly. In some cases it is thought that the unusually high temperature in the area of a varicocele may have a direct toxic effect upon the sperm-producing qualities of the testis. There are times when no adequate explanation seems to apply. Nevertheless, it seems to be the case that the presence of a varicocele can be associated with infertility. The degree of effect on sperm production and sperm quality is not necessarily related to the size of the varicocele. The varicocele may be small and yet the effect on fertility may be great. On physical examination, the male is examined while bearing down, very much as he would during a bowel movement, and the scrotum and testes are felt. The varicocele is described as feeling very much like a bag of worms. Because bearing down decreases the blood leaving these vessels, blood gathers in the swollen veins and the feeling is very much like that of a series of pulsating worms. The appropriate treatment for this is a surgical approach.

Another structural abnormality may be the absence or obstruction of the vas deferens and/or the epididymis, the conduits of sperm from the testes to the penis. In this case, sperm is being produced by the testis but the route that it must travel to the penis is blocked. This may be a result of a congenital abnormality, or may be a result of a purposeful surgical obstruction such as following a vasectomy for sterilization purposes. The epididymis adds fructose to the semen. If the semen analysis shows no sperm present and no fructose present, these findings are consistent with the absence or the obstruction of the vas deferens or the epididymis. If, on the other hand, no sperm are present but fructose can be found in the seminal fluid on masturbation, then one has a picture of a nonfunctioning testis but an open channel from the testes into the penis.

Absence of Vas Deferens and/or Epididymis

Another structural problem leading to infertility is *cryptorchidism*. Embryonically, the human male testes are found within the abdomen and should migrate into the scrotal sac by birth. Failure of the testes to descend into the scrotum is called cryptorchidism. This abnormal, intra-abdominal environment severely affects the development of the testes and if allowed to continue long enough can prevent normal sperm development. At the time a diagnosis of an undescended testis is made, con-

Cryptorchidism

sideration for surgical treatment to bring the testis into the scrotal sac should be considered. A biopsy of the testis will allow the patient and the physician to judge what the possibility is of the patient to produce a child in the future. The diagnosis of cryptorchidism can be made simply by examining the scrotal sac to see whether or not testes are present. This clinical state must be differentiated from *anorchia*, where the patient is born without testes. No testes are present either scrotally or intra-abdominally. For the patient with anorchia, there is no way of fathering a child, at this time.

It is possible for sperm upon entering the urethra, to go back into the bladder rather than extending forward into the penis. This is called *retrograde ejaculation*. Retrograde ejaculation may be a result of the effect of certain drugs or medications such as tranquilizers or antihypertensive medication. It may be a product of nerve degeneration or in rare cases may follow a prostatectomy The diagnosis can be made by the failure to find sperm being emitted from the penis but finding sperm in a urine sample voided immediately following a dry ejaculation. When this is a result of medication administered it can be treated by changing drugs or diminishing drug dose. When this is the result of other problems the patient may be treated by catheterizing the male after ejaculation and obtaining the sperm deposited within the bladder and using this for artificial insemination.

If the male's penis is abnormal in structure with a hole that is usually at its tip placed in an abnormal position, delivery of sperm within the vagina becomes very difficult. *Hypospadias*, a condition where the opening of the penis is on the underside,

Retrograde Ejaculation

Hypospadias

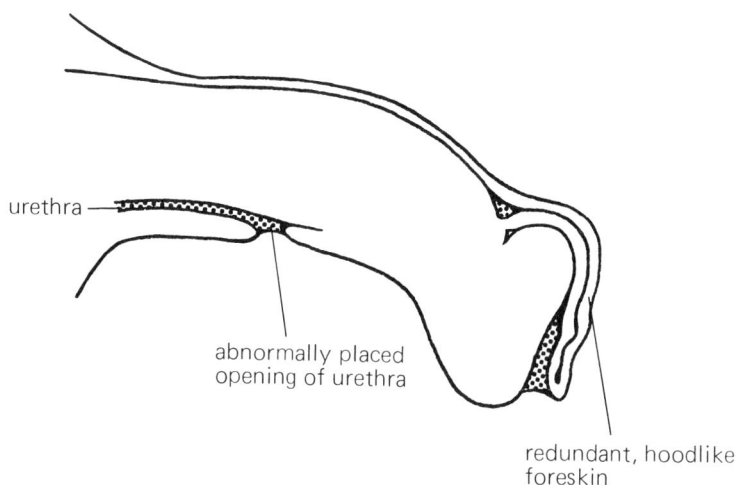

urethra

abnormally placed
opening of urethra

redundant, hoodlike
foreskin

Figure 4.2 *The opening of the urethra, the tube which carries urine and sperm, is in an abnormal position, away from the end of the penis on its underside. Because of its location, the normal placement of sperm within the vaginia may be prevented.*

back from the tip, is one of the more common forms of this abnormality. Instead of sperm being deposited within the vagina, next to the cervix, within the cervical mucus, it may be deposited in the outer third of the vagina so that an insufficient amount, if any, will ever reach the cervix. Therapy for this is simply to obtain a specimen of sperm by masturbation from the affected man and deliver it to the woman by artificial insemination. Since the sperm should be normal in every other respect, the probability of achieving success should be quite good. (See Figure 4.2.)

The next major category of the cause of male infertility is *infection.* Any process causing inflam- Infection mation of the testes may significantly damage the cells producing sperm. An inflammation of the testes is referred to as *orchitis*. When adult males

Mumps

contract mumps after puberty, approximately 25% sustain testicular damage which later reflects itself in reproductive problems. When a male develops an orchitis the testes become swollen and very painful to the touch. If a piece of tissue is removed from the testis at a later date microscopic examination shows definite irreversible damage to some of the sperm-producing elements and atrophy of the testis itself.

Gonorrhea

This damage is irreversible. Gonorrhea may also produce damage to the sperm producing elements of the testes. Prompt treatment for gonorrhea should be encouraged for both the prevention of epidemics and the maintenance of fertility of the affected patient.

T-mycoplasma

Another infectious agent, partway between a virus and a bacterium, is T-mycoplasma. Its role in infertility is still a product of much debate. Nevertheless, in at least some cases, T-mycoplasma seems to fasten itself to the sperm cells and render them less mobile and less capable of producing fertilization. The diagnosis of T-mycoplasma infection is very difficult to make. The ideal way would be to take a sample of semen and culture it to grow up the organism and thus demonstrate its presence. However, T-mycoplasma does not seem to cooperate and does not always grow very well in a laboratory culture medium. Furthermore, T-mycoplasma has also been found in patients with no reproductive problems at all. In years to come its role in infertility will be clarified.

Genetic

There are also genetic reasons for the inability of a male to cause a conception. Normal males have

Klinefelter's Syndrome

46 chromosomes with an X and a Y chromosome. Normal females have 46 chromosomes with two X

chromosomes, referred to as 46 XX. If an individual has an abnormal chromosomal composition, frequently their reproductive ability is compromised. If a male, instead of having XY sex chromosomes, has two XX chromosomes along with the Y resulting in an XXY chromosomal pattern, these males would be unable to reproduce in most cases. Physical examination shows a male with slightly widened hips and slightly longer than normal extremities. His breasts may be minimally enlarged and his testes small. A semen analysis will fail to show any sperm present and a biopsy of his testes will show no sperm. An XXY male is known as having *Klinefelter's Syndrome*. In some rare cases a man with Klinefelter's Syndrome can produce sperm but in numbers so small as to make producing pregnancy virtually impossible. Even though a male with this syndrome has an extra X chromosome, in areas other than reproduction he is a normal man and should not fear that he is a cross between a male and female.

The *hormonal* causes of male infertility include the malfunctioning of almost any of the glands of the endocrine system. If the pituitary gland is the cause of the infertility problem, it may be the result of one of two kinds of deficiencies. The male may have a selective deficiency of FSH and LH. These hormones are necessary for the development of sperm cells and for the production of *testosterone*, the hormone responsible for male secondary sex characteristics. If the pituitary gland produces all other hormones except FSH and LH it is said to have a selective deficiency of these hormones. One such clinical state is described as *Kallman's Syndrome* and is usually associated with coexisting

Hormonal

Kallman's Syndrome

61

defects in the sense of smell and occasionally in deformities of the face. Another possibility is that the pituitary gland may fail to produce almost all of its hormones, not just FSH and LH. The result is low or nonfunctioning of the testes, thyroid gland and the adrenal gland. This is called *pan-hypopituitarism*. The diagnosis of a selective FSH and LH deficiency or a pan-hypopituitarism can be made by drawing blood and testing it for levels of the pituitary hormones. Deficiencies of just FSH and LH make the diagnosis of a selective deficiency whereas total absence of all pituitary hormones makes the diagnosis of a pan-hypopituitarism problem. In the latter case physical examination shows signs consistent with thyroid and adrenal problems. It is also possible for the patient to have poor functioning of the thyroid or the adrenal gland unrelated to any pituitary problems.

Pan-hypopituitarism

Thyroid
Adrenal

The diagnosis of an underfunctioning of these two endrocrine glands can be made by studying the blood levels of thyroxine in the first case and cortisol in the second. Occasionally defects in the entire chemistry of the adrenal gland may exist. The diagnosis can be made by asking a patient to collect all the urine produced in a twenty-four-hour period and sending this urine for examination for the biochemical products of the adrenal gland. Assays are usually done for substances known as 17-hydroxycorticosteroids, 17-ketosteroids and pregnantriol.

Drugs

Drugs and medications can affect sperm production. Narcotics can affect the hypothalamic pituitary axis and prevent normal production of FSH and LH. With this, sperm production may diminish directly. Narcotics, alcohol, tranquilizers and certain kinds of antidepressant medication and antihypertensive medication may interfere with the ability to ejaculate and may be associated with retrograde ejaculation. Other drugs such as methotrexate, antimalarial drugs, nitrofurantoin, may be associated with defects in sperm cell production. Their effect may be found by simply doing a semen analysis. The resulting low sperm count, or in the case of retrograde ejaculation, the absence of sperm after apparent ejaculation but with sperm found in the urine specimen, helps make the diagnosis. Diminishing the dose or changing the medication will usually reverse the effects of the medication.

The environment plays a role in the cause of infertility. Radiation will affect any rapidly dividing cell population. Since the cells producing spermatazoa belong to this class, these cells may be quite sensitive to radiation damage. Following significant radiation it may take up to two years for the return of sperm cell production. It appears to be the case that if sperm cell production has not returned four years after radiation it probably will not return. Heat, applied locally around the testes can also affect sperm cell production. Men who spend most of their time sitting at the job such as truck drivers, taxi drivers and office desk workers tend to have a lower sperm count than the general population.

Infertility related to the female factor has several causes. The most common is infertility resulting from a failure to ovulate. This is called *anovulation*, literally non-ovulation. Anovulation can occur because the ovary has exhausted its supply of eggs and is now no longer functioning. This is called

Environment

II
FEMALE
FACTOR
Anovulation

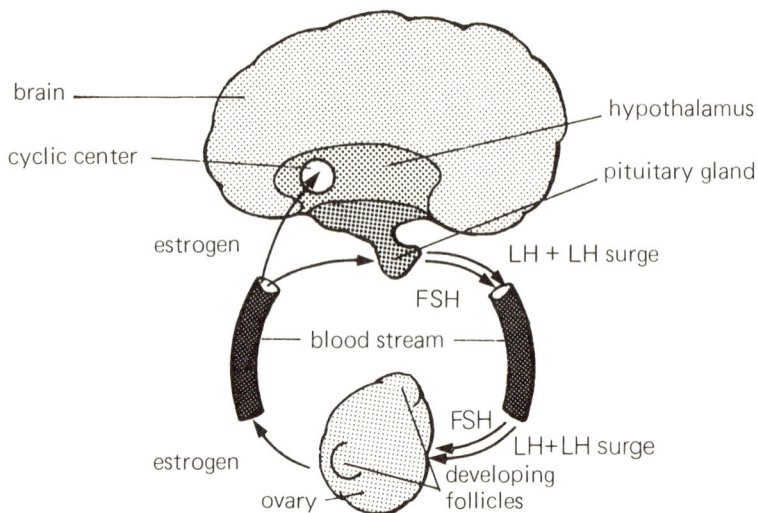

Figure 4.3 *Normal hypothalamus, pituitary gland and ovary interacting.*

Ovarian Failure *ovarian failure* and usually occurs in menopausal women in their mid-forties. When this occurs in a woman of younger age such as age twenty or thirty, it is called *premature ovarian failure*. Fortunately, if the woman has not had abdominal radiotherapy or surgical damage to both ovaries, premature ovarian failure is an uncommon cause of infertility. I say "fortunately" because there is no treatment at this time for documented premature ovarian failure. In order to confirm the fact that a woman has exhausted her supply of eggs, many physicians will take an ovarian biopsy, (surgically cutting a small section of the ovary), to confirm the diagnosis under the microscope. Hormonal studies, FSH and LH levels also may be used. (See Figures 4.3 and 4.4.)

The more common situation is for the ovary to be

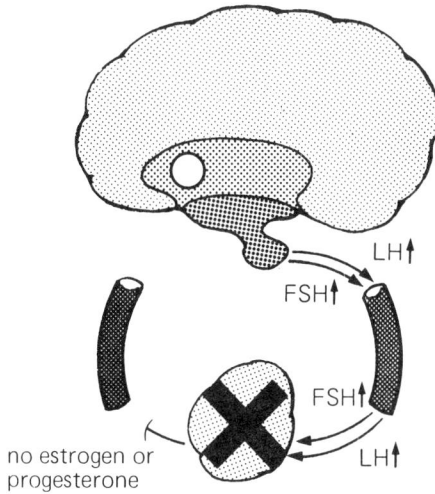

Figure 4.4 *Ovarian failure. The ovary fails to respond to FSH and LH stimulation. No estrogen or progesterone is produced. No ovulation occurs., Blood levels of FSH and LH are high. Blood studies: FSH and LH are high; Estrogen is almost absent.*

functioning but for there to be an insufficient hormonal stimulus to cause ovulation. FSH and LH are produced by the pituitary gland under the influence of the hypothalamus. A certain baseline amount of these hormones must be produced to stimulate and ready the ovary to ovulate. Then, at mid-cycle, with the specific stimulation of the hypothalamus, the pituitary releases a massive amount of FSH and LH, producing a sudden surge of these substances within the bloodstream. It is this surge of LH and FSH that produces ovulation . The baseline levels of FSH and LH ready the ovary for ovulation and cause it to produce its normal levels of estrogen. Following ovulation, these lower levels help to maintain the corpus luteum and allow the ovary to produce estrogen and progesterone.

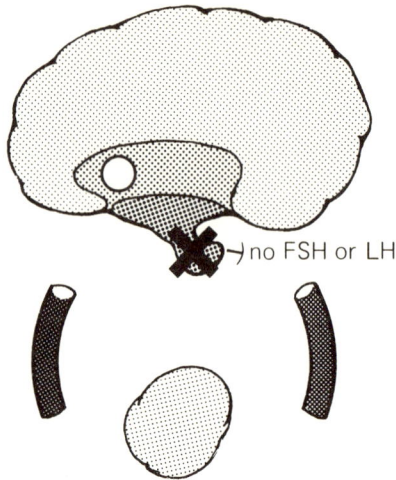

Figure 4.5 *Pituitary problem. No FSH and LH are produced. Therefore the ovary receives no stimulation. Thus, no estrogen or progesterone is made and no ovulation occurs. Blood studies: FSH and LH are almost absent; Estrogen is almost absent.*

Pituitary Problem

If the pituitary is unable to produce FSH and LH because of damage to the cells that make these hormones, then the stimulation to the ovary readying it for ovulation will not occur. The result is the patient with essentially no FSH and LH in her blood, little or no estrogen produced from her ovary and no ovulation. This patient has a pituitary problem as a cause of her lack of ovulation. (See Figure 4.5.)

Hypothalamic Problem

If a woman has a functioning ovary and pituitary, but has a hypothalamus that does not stimulate ovulation, the result would be FSH and LH produced in the usual baseline manner and estrogen produced from the ovary. No mid-cycle surge of the pituitary hormones would occur and there would be no ovulation. Studying a blood sample from such a patient would show normal

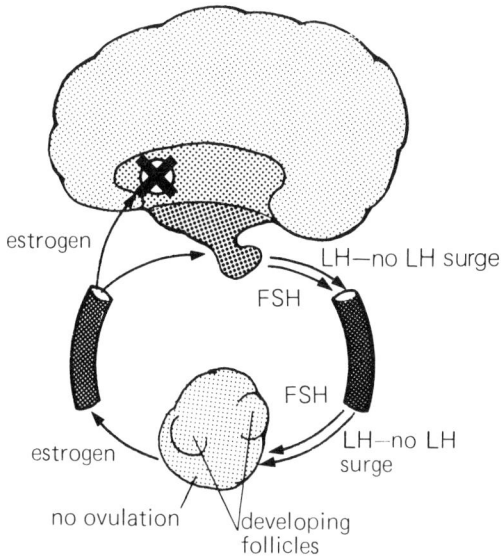

Figure 4.6 *Hypothalmic problem. FSH and LH are being produced, but no LH surge occurs. Since the LH surge is necessary for ovulation, no ovulation occurs.*
Blood studies: FSH and LH are of normal range; Estrogen is of normal range; Progesterone is absent.

levels of LH and FSH and normal levels of estrogen. This patient has a malfunctioning hypothalamus as the cause of her non-ovulation. (See Figure 4.6.)

I have just described three kinds of patients who do not ovulate. The first was a woman with premature ovarian failure. Her ovaries have exhausted their supply of eggs. She has a very high level of FSH and LH in her blood, low levels of estrogen and no ovulation. The second patient had a problem with her pituitary resulting in extremely low levels of FSH, LH and estrogen in her blood and no ovulation. The last patient had a malfunctioning of the cyclic center of her hypothalamus. She had normal levels of FSH, LH and estrogen in her blood and she, too, does not ovulate. Blood samples drawn from the arm of each of these patients will help to differentiate one from the other. Another way to determine the reason for the lack of ovulation is to administer progesterone or a progesterone-like drug to the patient. If she has hypothalamic anovulation, that is, if she is not ovulating because of a problem with her hypothalamus, progesterone administration will be followed by a menstrual period in several days. If she has pituitary or ovarian problems she will not have a menstrual period following progesterone.

Though these categories are described as distinct groups for the purpose of this book, it must be emphasized that in real life they may merge with one another. The physician may have to do tests well beyond the scope of this book to differentiate one kind of lack of ovulation from another.

Other Hormonal Problems Associated with Anovulation

The various organ systems of the human body interact and remain in balance with one another. It is not uncommon for a problem in one system to be reflected by an improper functioning of another organ system. This is the case with hypothalamic anovulation. Not infrequently hypothalamic anovulation may be a result of a glandular problem unassociated with the female reproductive system. An overfunctioning or an underfunctioning of the thyroid or adrenal gland, or an early diabetic state, may all first show themselves as a hypothalamic cause of non-ovulation.

A patient with hypothalamic anovulation may manage to ovulate two, three or even four times a year and need not cease ovulating altogether. Though this is better than producing no eggs at all, it is still not very much of a help to those who are seeking a pregnancy. This is because rather than having twelve opportunities for pregnancy in a year, there may be only two, three or four. Furthermore, with regular ovulation the time that the woman is releasing her egg can be predicted month after month. When a woman is ovulating irregularly, the time of ovulation is generally not known and the chances of having sexual relations at that time may be pure luck. So whether hypothalamic anovulation results in a total absence of the release of eggs or in an infrequent, irregular ovulation, both should be treated.

The second main category of causes of female infertility is that of hormonal causes that do not interfere with ovulation. In some cases the patient may have either an over- or under-activity of the thyroid or adrenal gland. The patient may have diabetes. In some cases this may affect ovulation but in other cases, the abnormal functioning may be so slight that ovulation does occur but pregnancy may not occur. It is not always obvious as to why this should happen. It may be that the patient becomes pregnant but then loses the pregnancy so quickly that a period is never missed. The pregnancy test never turns positive and the patient is never aware of the fact that she had become pregnant in the first place. Other patients become pregnant but, because of hormonal problems, lose their pregnancies several weeks after conception.

Hormonal Problems Unassociated with Anovulation

Thyroid
Adrenal
Diabetes

Progesterone, a hormone produced by the ovary after ovulation, is necessary for the survival of the newly fertilized egg. If progesterone is produced for too short a period of time, or in too small a quantity, the fertilized egg may not be able to survive. This is

Progesterone

Inadequate Luteal Phase frequently called an *inadequate luteal phase* or a *luteal phase defect*. This may be a cause of infertility in apparently normally ovulating women.

Some investigators feel that this may also be one of the causes of miscarriages in early pregnancy. Determining whether or not a hormonal deficiency exists is relatively simple. A sample of blood, and in some cases, urine, is collected and studied for the hormonal products of the gland being investigated. A screening test for diabetes can be made by studying the blood for blood sugar levels. In the event that the blood sugar level is abnormal, more detailed studies of sugar metabolism can be done utilizing a glucose tolerance test.

Structural Problems

The third major category of causes of infertility in the female is that of *structural abnormalities*. It is obvious that if a woman does not have a uterus or Fallopian tubes, or a vagina, that pregnancy, by ordinary means, is impossible. If a woman has had a previous inflammatory disease involving her Fallopian tubes as a result of gonorrhea or an acute appendicitis, it is possible that there may be scar tissue around the Fallopian tubes, possibly within the walls of the tubes, preventing their function, and partially obstructing the channel within the tube. Remember that in order for the Fallopian tube to function it must have the delicate, folded lining within a muscular tube that is capable of free movement. The tube must be capable of a coordinated contraction, moving the sperm in one direction, the egg in the other direction and the fertilized egg back toward the uterus. If a previous infectious process has caused scarring of the Fallopian tube, the delicate lining of the structure may have been irreversibly damaged. Muscle fibers within the wall

Absence of Uterus, Tubes or Vagina

Tubal Problems

Scarring

70

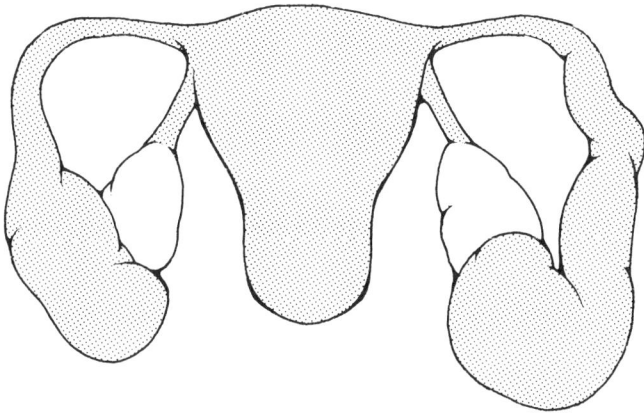

Figure 4.7 *Hydrosalpinx. Both tubes are closed and enlarged into two thin-walled, saclike structures. These tubes are unable to pick up an egg.*

may have been destroyed and replaced by fibrous scar tissue. This scar tissue is not capable of contracting and will upset the coordinated movement of the tube. The channel within the tube itself may develop scar tissue, which will grow and close off the tube.

The end of the Fallopian tube is a funnel-shaped, freely movable, highly specialized structure called the *fimbria*. It is designed to pick up the egg when it is released from the ovary. Its ability to move freely is an important factor in catching the egg. When the fimbria becomes inflamed, whether as a result of infection or irritation, the delicate folds may stick together. Instead of the end of the tube being open and funnel-shaped, it may be drawn together like the end of a laundry bag with its strings pulled tightly. In severe cases, the opening may be totally obliterated and the end of the tube may appear club-shaped. (See Figure 4.7.) When the end of the tube is completely obstructed, as a result of an infectious process such as gonorrhea, the entire Fallopian tube fills with pus and turns into a large sac. With time, the infectious process resolves but the sac with its scarring remains. The lining of the Fallopian tube may be permanently destroyed and the muscle within the wall replaced partially or completely with connective tissue. After the tube has healed instead of being filled with pus, it is filled with a sterile, clear fluid. This scarred, fluid filled sac-like tube, is a virtually nonfunctioning remnant of the previous Fallopian tube. The only way of remedying this is by attempting surgical reconstruction. This will be discussed more fully in the chapter on therapy.

Adhesion Formation

In an attempt to wall off an area of irritation, when an area of the abdomen is inflamed, the body produces layers of connective tissue to isolate the irritated area. These bands of connective tissue known as *adhesions*, may hold the Fallopian tube in such a position that, at later times, egg pickup becomes almost impossible and infertility results. (See Figure 4.8.)

Gonorrhea or a pelvic infection is not the only cause of adhesions around the tubes and ovaries. Any irritative process will result in a local tissue reaction, or inflammation which in some cases is followed by adhesion formation. Some women are much more susceptible to adhesion formation than others.

If a fluid filled ovarian cyst forms and breaks, the liquid that comes out may irritate the tissue covering the tubes and an adhesion may form. If the ovary bleeds excessively from an area where an egg was released, adhesions may follow. The use of an intrauterine contraceptive, an IUD, can be followed

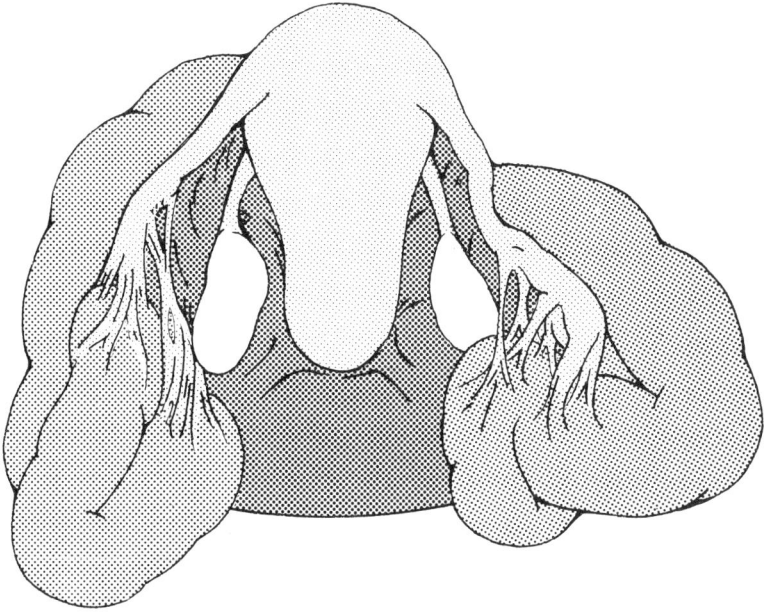

Figure 4.8 *Adhesions immobilizing the tube. Connective tissue bands (adhesions) may form around the Fallopian tubes preventing the fimbria from picking up an ovum or actually obstructing the tube.*

by tubal adhesion formation in some patients. Even a high fever, in experimental animals, causes a general reaction throughout the body followed by pelvic adhesions in some cases. This same thing may occur in humans. This may be important since almost every adult has had a high fever at some time during childhood. Once again, one is left with the feeling that it is not surprising that a particular woman has tubal adhesions but rather it is surprising that not every woman has them.

Endometriosis is another cause of tubal scarring. The lining of the uterus, the endometrium, is composed of actively growing tissue that expands

Endometriosis

73

during a woman's menstrual cycle and crumbles around the time of her period. For unknown reasons, some women have this tissue in other locations besides the cavity of the uterus. When this occurs it is called endometriosis. The ovaries, the outer surface of the Fallopian tubes, and the uterosacral ligaments on the back of the uterus are the most common locations for this misplaced endometrium. When these areas of endometriosis expand during the cycle they become very sensitive to the touch. If, during sexual activities, these areas are shaken or touched, they usually produce significant pain. The result is painful sexual relations or *dyspareunia*. (See Figure 4.9.)

During the time of the menses the areas of endometriosis may crumble and produce a pasty material that is extremely irritating to the surrounding tissues. This results in severe pain during menses which is called *dysmenorrhea*. This irritating material may actually destroy some of the tissue around it. As the area heals, fibrous, connective tissue replaces the damaged tissue and a scar is formed. The area around this becomes inflamed and later adhesions form. The end product of this is a Fallopian tube with areas of muscle destroyed and scarred that is held in an abnormal position by adhesions. There are many degrees of endometriosis. In some cases there may be areas that are so small that they would escape observation by all but the most diligent physician with little scarring and no adhesions. In other cases the areas may produce masses that are so large that the entire lower abdomen is filled. It is interesting that infertility may result in patients with even the smallest areas of endometriosis that are well away

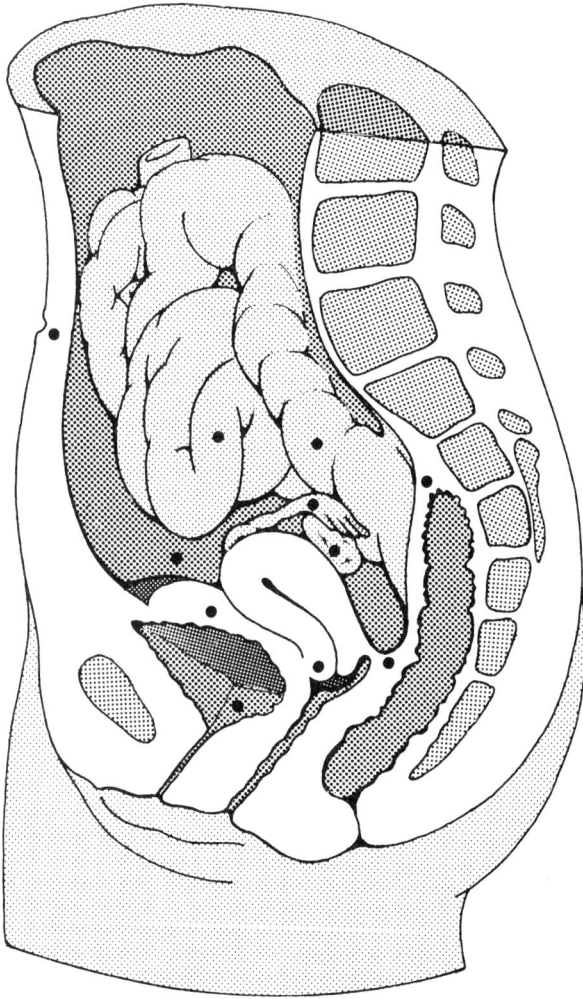

Figure 4.9 *Endometriosis. Some of the possible sites of
endometriosis are shown.*

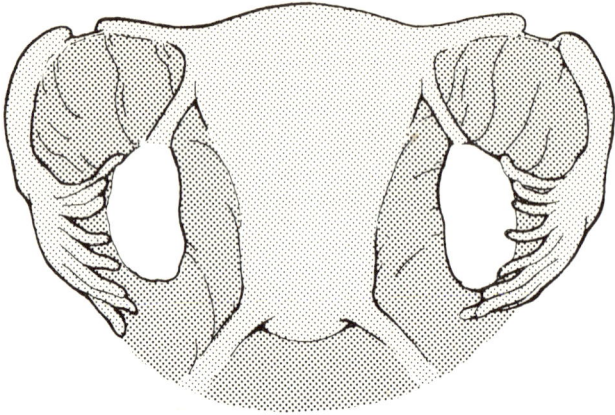

Figure 4.10 *Tubal ligation (sterilization). Small segments of the middle of the tubes have been removed.*

from the tubes and ovaries.

Endometriosis is usually treatable by medication and/or surgery. This will be discussed in a subsequent chapter.

Connective tissue may form over the surface of the ovary. In a healed state, that is, after an inflammatory process has subsided, the connective tissue remains. This connective tissue actively prevents the egg from escaping from the surface of the ovary thus preventing its pickup by the fimbria of the Fallopian tube. The only way of correcting this is by surgically removing the connective tissue. This too will be discussed in a subsequent chapter.

Previous Sterilization

Another cause of infertility may be a previous sterilization procedure. A tubal ligation may have been done where a segment of the Fallopian tube has been removed and the two free ends of the tube healed closed. The result is a double obstruction within the channel of the Fallopian tube preventing

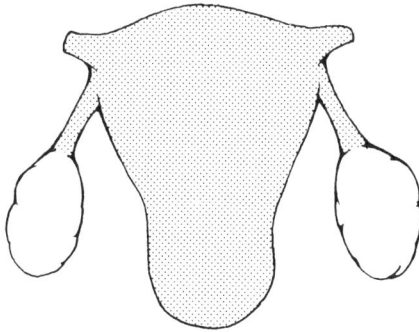

Figure 4.11 *Tubal sterilization. Here the entire tubes have been removed. This is known as a* salpingectomy.

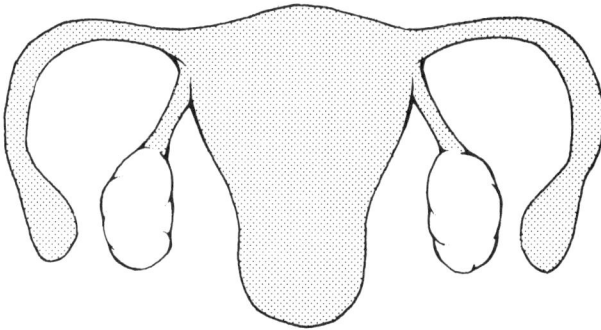

Figure 4.12 *Tubal sterilization. Here the fimbria have been removed from both tubes. This is known as a* fimbriectomy.

the movement of the egg and the sperm so that they may not reach one another. If the woman now desires pregnancy the only way of remedying this is by surgically reconnecting the tubes. It is also possible that in an attempt to produce permanent sterilization, the initial surgeon removed the entire Fallopian tube or the segment containing the fimbria. If this is the case, with the available surgical techniques at this time, there is no way of replacing or reconstructing such a tube and restoring fertility. (See Figures 4.10, 4.11, 4.12.)

There are various kinds of surgical sterilization available today. In the chapter on therapy the potential for reversibility of these surgical procedures will be discussed.

Uterine Problems Infertility may also result because of an abnormality in the structure of the uterine cavity. This may be a wall (or *septum*) extending down into the cavity or the deformity of the cavity by a benign tumor called a leiomyoma or in more conventional language, a *fibroid*. Occasionally, the front and back walls of the uterine cavity may have become stuck together. This may be the result of a previous infectious process or scarring of the uterine cavity. The front and back walls of the cavity become adherent to each other by the formation of scar tissue very much like the scar tissue previously discussed which may form around the Fallopian tubes. The presence of this scar tissue, obliterating the cavity, was first described by Asherman and is referred to as *Asherman's Syndrome*. (See Figures 4.13 and 4.14.)

An abnormality of the uterine cavity may be demonstrated using a *hysterosalpingogram*, that is, an x-ray of the uterine cavity, or by placing a specialized telescope called a *hysteroscope* in the uterine cavity through the cervix and actually visualizing the contents of the cavity.

Most frequently, abnormalities of the uterine cavity, other than Asherman's Syndrome, usually show their effect not by preventing pregnancy but by hindering the development of a pregnancy causing spontaneous abortion or a miscarriage. When a patient presents a history of pregnancy with

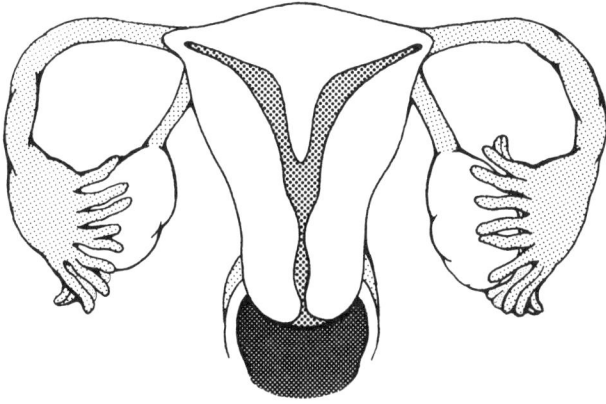

Figure 4.13 *Uterus with a septum.*

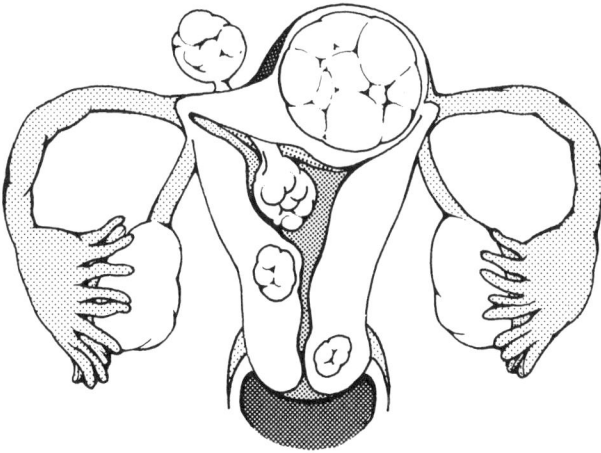

Figure 4.14 *Fibroids. These noncancerous tumors distort the surface of the uterus or may actually compress and close off the Fallopian tubes. In this way they may result in infertility or miscarriage.*

repeated loss of the pregnancy, the possibility of an intrauterine abnormality must be considered.

Cervical Structural Problems

The fourth kind of structural abnormality that may exist in the female reproductive tract is something called an *incompetent cervix*. The opening to the uterus, which is found at the inner most part of the vagina, is called the *cervix*. It has circular muscle and connective tissue running up into the body of the uterus and around the opening of the uterus, very much like the draw-strings on a laundry bag or sack. Once a patient becomes pregnant, the pregnancy grows within the cavity of the uterus and when the female stands up in the ordinary, every day walking position, the weight of the pregnancy is exerted downward against the cervix. It is the job of this connective tissue to keep the opening of the cervix closed until the time for labor is reached. If these fibers do not do their job, the cervix will gradually open as the weight of the growing pregnancy is exerted against it. Sometime in midpregnancy, the patient will suddenly feel a splash, or gush of some fluid and the pregnancy will be passed painlessly. This is unlike other kinds of miscarriage where the patient will feel cramps and the discomfort very much like real labor. Miscarriages associated with an incompetent cervix are most commonly painless.

Cervical Functional Problems

A fourth major category of the causes of infertility in the female is that of the improper functioning of the cervix. In order for sperm to enter the uterine cavity and the Fallopian tube, to fertilize the ovum, the sperm must swim through a large quantity of watery mucus secreted by the cervix. It is the function of this mucus to act as a medium through which the sperm may swim to reach the uterine cavity and the Fallopian tube. Some women produce too little cervical mucus. Others produce cervical mucus that is so thick that sperm cannot penetrate it. In either case, instead of the cervical mucus acting as a means through which the sperm may reach the uterine cavity and the egg, the cervical mucus acts as a barrier. The diagnosis of this can be made fairly simply by doing a *post-coital test*, sometimes called a *Simms-Huhner test*, at the time of ovulation. It is at this time that the cervical mucus should be present in its greatest volume and in its most favorable quality to support the life of the sperm. If a small quantity is found or if the texture of the mucus is thick rather than watery, the diagnosis of poor quality cervical mucus is made.

Thus far, male factors and female factors have been reviewed. The next major category in the causes of infertility is what I will call the problems in *male-female interaction.* In order for pregnancy to be established, a man and woman must have sexual relations, at least once and, ideally, several times around the time of ovulation for several cycles in succession. One should not begin to be concerned until the couple has had intercourse regularly for one year without the production of a pregnancy. If a couple is having relations less frequently or having intercourse at the wrong time of the cycle, the pregnancy cannot occur. The only way to determine whether or not this is occurring is for the physician to take a very careful history at the very first visit. It is for this reason that it is imperative that both the man and woman be present together at the first visit to the physician's office for an infertility evaluation. The history obtained will review the frequency, the technique and the timing of sexual relations.

**III
MALE-FEMALE
INTERACTION**

**Problems in
Timing
Intercourse**

**Problems in
Mechanics of
Intercourse**

Penis

Vagina

There are also certain social and cultural problems. For example, Orthodox Jews cannot have relations for one week after the cessation of a woman's menstrual flow. If the woman ovulates on cycle day fourteen and her menses go past cycle day eight, then intercourse will never occur at the time of ovulation and pregnancy cannot occur. Such factors must be taken into account in evaluating the problems of an infertile couple.

Another problem in male-female interaction is that of the actual mechanics of having intercourse. It is possible that the man is unable to obtain sufficient rigidity of his penis to penetrate the vagina of his female sex partner. It is also possible that the muscle tone and the tension of the woman is such that she constricts her vagina and penetration of her vagina by a normal penis is impossible. In either event, the result is that the male cannot deposit his sperm within the vagina of the female. Occasionally, when vaginal tone is maintained to such a degree that vaginal entrance is impossible, called *vaginismus*, the man may place his penis within the urethral opening of the woman. The urethra is the tube which drains the bladder and so is the opening through which urine flows when a woman urinates. If this opening is the area of least resistance, then it is possible to have urethral intercourse instead of vaginal intercourse. This is extremely unusual, but nevertheless it must be considered. Similarly, it is possible to have rectal intercourse when entrance into the vagina cannot be accomplished. On occasion, the couple may have had regular rectal intercourse without realizing it. When a man, who is known to have good semen specimens, and a woman are asked to have intercourse so a post-coital test can be done and no sperm is found within the vagina, then a problem of sexual technique seems very likely. One of the problems just outlined must be considered as a possibility. The remedy frequently involves further education, investigation of sexual techniques and occasionally, sex therapy. The results of this are excellent.

Another problem fitting under the general **Antibodies** category of male-female interaction is that of *antibodies.* If a man and a woman are having intercourse properly and non-moving sperm cells are found within the cervical mucus, the physician must consider that there is something within the cervical mucus or within the man's seminal fluid that is killing the sperm. One possible explanation for this is that the body's defense system, known as its immunological system, may be attacking the sperm and killing it.

The human body has a very special defense system. It can recognize which cells belong to that body and which cells belong to something or somebody else. Any cells that are foreign, i.e., do not belong to that particular individual, are recognized as potential invaders and are attacked. This works out rather well if the cell that is attacked is a disease causing micro-organism. The cells are attacked by covering them with a thin layer of antibodies made by the body, known as *gamma globulin.*

This renders the cells inactive and prepares them for destruction by other specialized cells of the body. Occasionally this defense system makes an error. Cells that are part of that individual's body may be recognized as foreign and may be attacked anyway. The result is a partial breakdown of the organ system to which the attacked cells belong. If the attacked cells are part of the surface of a joint, then the patient may develop arthritis. If the cells being attacked belong to the lungs, then the patient develops asthma.

Occasionally, though rarely, a male may become sensitive or allergic to his own sperm cells. In this case, he would produce sperm in normal numbers that may or may not move around when examined under the microscope but are unable to fertilize an egg because they are coated with gamma globulin. In another case a woman may produce antibodies to sperm cells. These antibodies may be in the blood, cervical mucus or in the secretions within the uterine cavity. When normal sperm interacts with the secretions containing antibodies the sperm cells are covered with gamma globulin and rendered inactive.

The post-coital tests in such cases may show reduced or total absence of movement of the sperm cells when studied. It is also possible that though each sperm cell is covered with gamma globulin, its movement is not reduced, only its ability to fertilize an egg. The post-coital test would then be normal but fertilization would still be impossible. Fortunately, this paradoxical situation is extremely unusual. Thus, if a post-coital test is normal and all other studies fail to show a cause for a couple's infertility, immunological studies to reveal anti-sperm antibodies in the male or in the female are still indicated.

Toxic Environment

In a certain sense, the immunological system, the defense system of the body, mistakenly may create a toxic environment for the sperm cell, making it impossible for the sperm cells to fertilize an egg.

Some investigators feel that other things may cause a toxic environment. In some cases the environment can be so bad as to actually kill the sperm cells. A micro-organism identified as the T-strain of mycoplasma has been incriminated as a possible culprit. This micro-organism has been found in the cervical mucus and the seminal fluid of couples with unexplained infertility or recurrent miscarriage. Unfortunately, it also has been found in couples with normal reproductive histories. Nevertheless, in some couples, when appropriate antibiotic therapy has been given and the organisms eradicated, fertility returns. The diagnosis is made by taking cervical mucus from the woman and seminal fluid from the man and adding it to a culture medium that will allow the micro-organism to grow. If the organism is seen on culture then the diagnosis is made and antibiotic therapy given. The significance of T-strain mycoplasma in infertility must still be clarified but this remains a significant area of investigation.

The fourth main category of causes of infertility is that of psychological causes. Though this may not be a significant problem at the outset of the infertility workup and treatment, psychological problems may become significant later on. Once the problems of a particular couple are identified and therapy has begun, an effort is made to determine as precisely as possible when ovulation occurs so the couple may have intercourse at that time and maximize their probability of achieving pregnancy. The result is that not infrequently the couple is sent home with a schedule of recommended times for sexual activity. Asking a man and woman to have sexual intercourse, month after month at precise,

IV PSYCHO-LOGICAL FACTOR

85

predetermined times places a great deal of stress on both partners. An activity that initially should represent the ultimate in human pleasures, may be reduced to a mechanical act or even a drudgery. The result may be the inability of the male to ejaculate, to release his sperm on the days required, or so much tension on the part of the woman that penile entrance into the vagina becomes impossible. Stress, whether the result of the outside world such as business pressures, etc., or a result of attempting pregnancy, may affect the male as well as the female. In the male, through the hormonal system, the sperm count and motility may be reduced. And as previously described, the ability to sexually perform may be hampered.

In the female, severe stress may turn off the ovulatory mechanism. In a school dormitory, at the time of mid-term and final examinations, many girls who have had regular menses up to this point, suddenly find that they have missed their periods. This is usually a result of the turning off of ovulation under a stress situation. Exactly the same thing may occur in a couple attempting pregnancy. Though the woman may never have had an ovulatory problem before, after all problems are corrected and a pregnancy is now attempted, she may cease ovulating thus adding an additional problem. Fortunately, this can be treated as any other ovulatory problem can be.

Stress may also effect the coordinated movement of the Fallopian tubes. Though this is much more controversial, it appears that under certain *very limited* circumstances tension may make the movement of the tubes that would allow the egg to be transported in one direction and the sperm in another, discoordinated. The lack of proper tubal movement, pickup of the egg and its movement toward the uterus may be hampered thus leading to infertility. I must emphasize that as our knowledge of other factors in infertility increases, the number of times one must use the psychological cause as an explanation diminishes. This is probably of minimal significance in the total picture of infertility.

Telling a man or a woman that they are actively causing their own infertility by worrying about their lack of success creates a self-defeating situation. It creates guilt where little or none may have existed before. Warning someone that she must not worry or else she will not become pregnant is like saying "do not think about your breathing." After you warn a person not to think in a certain manner, they cannot help thinking in precisely that manner. Other than heightening anxiety and making sexual performance difficult it is not even clear that the psychological factor is truly important in most infertile couples.

The next to the last category in the list of causes of infertility is that of genetic abnormalities. It is possible for the genetic material produced in an egg or a sperm cell to be defective. The usual result is that fertilization does not take place. A defective sperm cell rarely works and a defective ovum usually cannot be fertilized. If fertilization does occur and a defective structure is produced, there is usually early miscarriage.

**V
GENETIC
FACTOR**

Repeated spontaneous miscarriage, unrelated to hormonal and structural problems in the female, requires a genetic evaluation of both of the partners. Blood is drawn from both the male and the female and genetic studies are done on the cells obtained from these samples. Several weeks are required for this study. Genetic problems unfortunately are not treatable at this time. However, given the information that can be obtained from genetic studies, the couple can plan their future realistically, based on more complete information.

VI
INFERTILITY
OF UNDETER-
MINED
CAUSE

The last category is that of infertility of undetermined cause. At this time this represents one of the greatest challenges to the infertility specialist. This category is composed of a small number of couples in whom all adequate studies have been completed and no reason for the infertility has been found. Note that I have not said that these patients are normal. These couples are not told that "there is nothing wrong with you," or that "it is all in your head so go home and keep trying." As long as a man and a woman cannot accomplish what other couples can, they cannot be thought of as having nothing wrong with them. It is just that our tests may not be sensitive enough or sophisticated enough to find the problem. We, the specialists in Reproductive Medicine, are not yet smart enough to know all the possible causes and cures of infertility and therefore, we do not know the answer for these particular patients. The one thing that is clear is that as the specialty of Reproductive Endocrinology and Infertility advances, month by month, year by year, the percentage of patients with "infertility of undetermined cause" becomes smaller and smaller. Since we are not able to find the cause of this group's problems we are not able to treat them. Therefore, it is encouraging that as our knowledge expands, the number of people who fit into this category decreases and more and more patients are being helped.

Now that the theoretical reasons for infertility have been described, the next logical step is to determine which cause (or causes) applies to a particular couple. The next chapter will discuss infertility testing and give you insight into this area.

Chapter 5

Infertility Tests

THE TESTS TO DETERMINE the reason for
childlessness at first seem like a meaningless
obstacle course that two human beings must endure
before a physician can give them the reason for their
problem and begin therapy. The procedures become
much more difficult to endure because frequently,
by necessity, they are distributed over several weeks
or months. Some tests are somewhat uncomfortable, most are not. Nevertheless, understanding
why each procedure must be done and why it must
be done at a certain time makes it a bit easier to
tolerate. The purpose of this chapter is to discuss the
most commonly used tests in an infertility evaluation, to tell you how they are done, why they are
done, why they are done when they are done and
what kind of information you can expect from them.

I
GENERAL
TESTS

One of the most helpful studies done during the
course of an infertility evaluation is not a recently
discovered biochemical test. It does not require the
use of expensive equipment. It is simple, painless
and does not take weeks to provide information. It
is accomplished simply by talking with your
physician and answering his detailed questions. The

Initial
Interview

initial interview by your physician allows him to

obtain an extensive history from both members of the couple. This history will provide basic clues to the origin of the infertility.

An important first question is "how long have you been attempting pregnancy." This is asked to establish whether or not the couple has had a sufficient opportunity to achieve pregnancy. Eighty percent of those couples who will establish a pregnancy do so in one year. Based on this it has been decided that if a couple has had regular intercourse, for one year without achieving pregnancy, the man and woman are considered to have an infertility problem. By regular intercourse, I mean sexual activity at least every other day at the time of ovulation, or every week for twelve months.

The second general group of questions involves past reproductive performance. Has the female partner ever been pregnant before? If she has, how did the pregnancies end – with the birth of a live, healthy baby at term or with a miscarriage? Has the man ever fathered a pregnancy? Were these pregnancies with the same partner as now or with someone else?

Specific questions directed toward each member of the couple will explore the possible reasons for infertility more completely. Does the woman have regular periods with cramping? If she does, the chances that she is ovulating are very high. Irregular, painless menses that come as a complete surprise to the woman are usually not associated with ovulation. Though this is not an absolute rule, it does indicate some possibilities that require particular attention in the infertility studies. Does the woman feel one-sided, lower abdominal cramping or discomfort around the time of mid-cycle?

This is called *mittleschmertz* and refers to the cramping feeling associated with ovulation. The regular presence of mittleschmertz is further indication that ovulation is probably occurring. It should be pointed out that many women who ovulate regularly never feel this discomfort. The presence of mittleschmertz makes the occurrence of ovulation likely, while its absence means nothing.

The history obtained by the physician can rule out major causes of Fallopian tube scarring. Has the woman ever had abdominal surgery of any kind? Has she ever had gonorrhea or any pelvic infections? Did she have an infection of her uterus after an abortion or the birth of her last child? Though a woman may have no reason for tubal adhesions based on her past history, adhesions may still be present. The history obtained by your physician can only tell him that certain things are likely, not that they do not exist at all.

The male partner is questioned about previous surgery to his penis or testes. He is asked if he ever had an infection of his testes. Has he had the mumps as an adult? Has he ever had gonorrhea? The physician will ask about occupational or environmental factors. Is your job or life in general a stressful one? Are you exposed to pesticides, paints, solvents, cleaning fluids, high temperatures or radiation? All or these factors may decrease sperm production and motility.

What kind of underwear do you wear? Anything that increases the temperature of the testes such as briefs or tight tennis shorts will provide an unfavorable environment for sperm production and this results in a lowered sperm count and motility. Occasionally changing underwear from briefs to boxer shorts can make a significant improvement in sperm quality. It must be emphasized that it takes about ninety days for an improvement to be seen. Tight underwear is not the only way of elevating the temperature of the testes. Sitting for long periods of time as an office desk worker, cab driver or truck driver will accomplish the same thing.

Do you use any medication? Tranquilizers and drugs used to treat high blood pressure are two examples of drugs that can decrease sperm production or make ejaculation (the release of sperm by the penis) difficult. Do you use lubricants, such as petroleum jelly, when having intercourse? Almost all lubricants decrease sperm movement and therefore make the sperm cells less effective.

Are you on any special diets? An unusually drastic reduction in calories can affect sperm quality. Other questions to investigate a history of diabetes, thyroid disease and adrenal diseases in each member of the couple and their families are asked.

It would be impossible to review all that a complete infertility history covers. These examples are presented so that you can see what information can be obtained simply by talking with your doctor and answering his questions.

The initial interview is more than an opportunity for the doctor to obtain information. It is also an excellent time for you to ask questions. This is important because only by doing this, will you have an opportunity to satisfy your curiosity and to expose your fears. Incidentally, it is very rare for the facts to be as frightening as the fears carried by most patients. The interview should not be a unidirectional communication with the physician asking the questions and the man and woman answering them. Rather, this first meeting should be an easy interchange among all three people. Each member of the group asks and answers questions. In this way a rapport can be established and the basis for further and continuous communication and proper treatment is established.

Because nervousness in the physician's office, a common, normal reaction, can make it difficult to think of the questions that have been plaguing you for weeks and months, it is helpful to write down your questions and thoughts before coming for the initial interview. It may also be helpful to take notes in the doctor's office to help you remember his instructions and responses to your key questions. Though some people feel self-conscious about doing this, there is no reason to feel that way. You are going to a physician for help and you should do everything possible to move toward success.

Physical Examination

Routine Laboratory Tests

Following the interview a complete physical examination is performed. Routine screening blood tests are frequently obtained on the first visit. It is only after this, during subsequent visits, that the specialized infertility studies are carried out.

II SPECIALIZED TESTS

Specialized infertility tests can be divided into four general categories. The first is an evaluation of the male. The second is the determination of whether or not ovulation occurs in the female. The third is the determination of the architecture of the female reproductive system. Lastly, the fourth is an evaluation of the sperm within the female reproductive tract.

Even though, while in the process of evaluating a couple, a reason for infertility is discovered, the remainder of the workup should still be completed.

94

In some cases more than one reason for infertility might exist. If in the process of evaluation it is discovered that a woman is not ovulating, it is still possible that she may have an obstruction of one or both Fallopian tubes and/or her husband may have poor sperm. If one were to stop the evaluation at the point where it was discovered the woman is not ovulating, and one were to treat the patient for that alone, the other problems would not be discovered and pregnancy would not occur. Thus, barring some special circumstances, the entire infertility evaluation should be completed regardless of the findings during the progress of the workup. It must be emphasized however, that in medicine as in many other things, no rules are absolute.

Evaluation of the male is relatively simple. The male is asked to produce a semen specimen by masturbation, deposit it into a clean glass jar and deliver it to a laboratory for evaluation within two hours of the production of the specimen. For males who are unable to masturbate, the specimen may be collected by having sexual relations and withdrawing the penis from the vagina just prior to the release of the sperm and releasing the sperm into a glass container. In other cases, where withdrawal of the penis cannot be accomplished in time, a special plastic condom may be used. The sperm so collected may then be brought to the laboratory for analysis. Unfortunately, the materials out of which condoms are constructed, and sometimes the chemicals used to line condoms may affect the sperm and can damage or kill some of the sperm cells producing an artificially poor specimen when analyzed. If the choice is between getting a specimen by this manner or no way at all then the

Male Factor Evaluation (First Basic Group of Tests)

Semen Analysis

95

use of a condom under certain circumstances may be making the best of a poor situation.

When the specimen reaches the laboratory the total volume of the fluid is measured. The number of sperm cells per unit volume is counted and reported to the doctor. The sperm cells themselves are then studied. Not all sperm produced are of normal shape nor are all the sperm cells moving. It is only the normal, moving sperm cells that are capable of producing pregnancy. Therefore, it is important to evaluate the specimen for the percent of sperm cells that are of normal shape and that are found to be moving. The moving sperm cells are described as *motile* sperm cells. And so after the number of sperm is counted, a slide is made and the percent of all sperm cells that are moving and the percent of all sperm cells of normal shape, are recorded. The physician thus receives a report stating the volume of fluid presented, the number of sperm cells per unit volume of fluid, the percent of normal forms seen and the percent of motile, or moving, forms seen. All of these factors are important in determining the ability of the male partner to produce a pregnancy. Different laboratories have different normal values for their particular technicians using their particular counting and dilution techniques. It is important when reading a given laboratory report to know what the normal values are for that particular laboratory.

The semen sample should also be checked for fructose levels. Fructose is a sugar which is added to the seminal fluid by the epididymis. If the semen analysis fails to show any sperm present it is not known whether the testis has failed to produce sperm or if normal sperm has been produced but it cannot reach the penis because of an obstruction in the path to the penis. By analyzing the sample for fructose levels one can differentiate between these two conditions. If no sperm is present but fructose is found one knows that the epididymis is present in that patient and that its secretions have found their way up through the vas deferens, out through the urethra and opening of the penis. If, on the other hand, no fructose is found then a possibility of a congenital absence of the epididymis or an obstruction of the vas deferens must be considered. In this latter situation it is possible that the testis is making sperm but because of an obstruction in its pathway, it cannot reach the penis and the outer world.

To further evaluate the patient who is *azospermic*, that is, produces no sperm, the physician will consider removing a small sliver of the testis and studying it under the microscope. This procedure, called a *testicular biopsy*, is done under   Testicular Biopsy
anesthesia and is reserved to determine whether or not an azospermic patient is indeed producing sperm within his testes. If sperm cells are seen on biopsy then it is apparent that the azospermic male has an obstruction somewhere in the system connecting the testes to the penis. If no sperm cells are seen then particular attention is directed to the kind of microscopic anatomy seen. Frequently, this will give clues to appropriate medical therapy that may assist in improving a man's fertility.

Another test that is used to evaluate the azo-   Vasography
spermic male is an x-ray procedure to visualize the pathway from the testes to penis to assure that it is open and unobstructed. The procedure, called *vasography*, is done by putting a tube into the vas deferens and injecting dye. If x-rays are taken at this

time, the path of the dye through this structure can be seen and a point of obstruction, if it exists, can be pinpointed. It must be noted that these studies are reserved for azospermic or severely oligospermic males, men who have very little or absolutely no sperm in their ejaculates.

Homonal Studies

If an endocrine problem is being considered, blood is drawn for FSH and LH levels and for thyroid studies and a twenty-four hour urine sample may be collected for 17-hydroxysteroid, 17-ketosteroid and pregnantriol levels.

Female Factor Evaluation

Ovulation Determination (Second Basic Group of Tests)

The second group of tests I mentioned involve the female. These include studies that determine whether or not ovulation occurs. If we were to sit down and attempt to devise a way of figuring out if a woman is making eggs it would be helpful to figure out something that happens after the production and the release of an egg that is not found under ordinary circumstances. When we think about it, it becomes apparent that the hormone progesterone is produced after ovulation and is not produced before or without ovulation. Progesterone has the ability to raise the temperature of a woman and to cause certain changes in the lining of the uterus. The

Basal Body Temperature

simplest test for ovulation is simply taking one's temperature, orally or rectally, the first thing in the morning, before getting out of bed, before beginning any activity. The reason this is important is because any movement after arising requires the release of energy by the body and therefore, the elevation of the resting temperature. The temperature recorded first thing in the morning, before any activity, is more uniform and will reflect the presence or absence of progesterone more clearly. Each morning, the first thing upon arising, the woman

98

measures her temperature and records it on a temperature chart next to the particular day of her cycle, calling the first day of her menses, cycle day one.

When all the dots on the temperature chart are connected, if ovulation has occurred, that part of the temperature chart following ovulation will show an elevation and a flat, straight line until just prior to menses. With the onset of menses or perhaps a day earlier, the woman's temperature will fall back to her pre-ovulatory levels. It is important to realize that the level of the temperature does not reflect the amount of progesterone produced. Nor can one determine precisely when ovulation occurs from the temperature curve. One can merely have the impression of a particular interval of several days during which time ovulation probably has occurred. (See Figure 5.1.)

Classically, the temperature curve around the time of ovulation shows a dip, then a gradual rise and a plateau lasting approximately fourteen days. Ovulation may occur anywhere from the dip to the rise, to the beginning of the plateau. It is impossible to determine while the curve is occurring, that is during the menstrual cycle, exactly what day ovulation has occurred based on the shape of the curve.

The advantages of the basal body metabolism chart are that measuring temperature is an inexpensive and a painless procedure. However, the test is basically a crude one and the information generated somewhat unreliable. There are some patients who have demonstrated that they ovulate as by various tests but who do not produce a temperature curve consistent with ovulation. There are others where the rising part of the curve occurs over a several day

i. Advantage

ii. Disadvantage

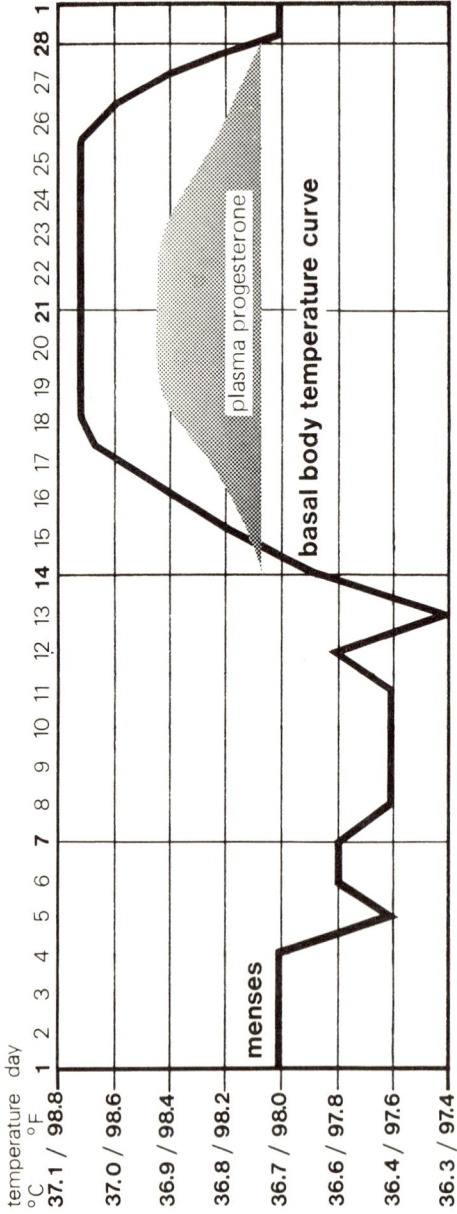

Figure 5.1 *Basal body temperature. When a woman's temperature is measured immediately upon awakening and this is charted according to the day of the menstrual cycle, one gets a basal body temperature curve. The hormone progesterone, which is produced only after ovulation, makes a woman's basal temperature rise. Thus, if ovulation has occurred, the basal body temperature curve will show a rise and a plateau after ovulation. Note that the rise and fall in basal temperature somewhat parallels the rise and fall of progesterone levels.*

period. You need not get terribly disturbed if your own basal body temperature curve does not resemble the classic ones in the textbooks. The only information one should attempt to get from a temperature curve is preliminary information confirming that ovulation occurs and to determine the approximate time, within a several day period, of when it occurred in past cycles.

Progesterone causes certain changes in the structure of the tissue lining the uterus. The changes are so regular and predictable that it is possible to look at a piece of tissue taken from the lining of the uterus and by looking at its structure, determine how many days earlier ovulation had occurred. We can utilize this as a more accurate test of ovulation. By taking the basal body temperature curve we have an approximate idea of when the woman released an egg. We then count several days thereafter and take a sample of the tissue lining the uterus. The tissue is then sent to a physician who specializes in evaluating the microscopic structure of tissue, a pathologist, and he tells us whether or not the tissue is consistent with ovulation and if so, how many days earlier ovulation has occurred. This procedure is called an *endometrial biopsy*. Biopsy means the removal of tissue for examination.

Endometrial Biopsy

For an endometrial biopsy, a woman is asked to position herself on the examining table as she would for an ordinary pelvic examination. The physician then, gently, inserts a speculum into the patient's vagina in order to visualize the cervix. The vagina is cleaned with cotton moistened with an antiseptic liquid. Up to this point the sensations felt by the woman are almost identical to those associated with a routine Pap smear examination. Next, the

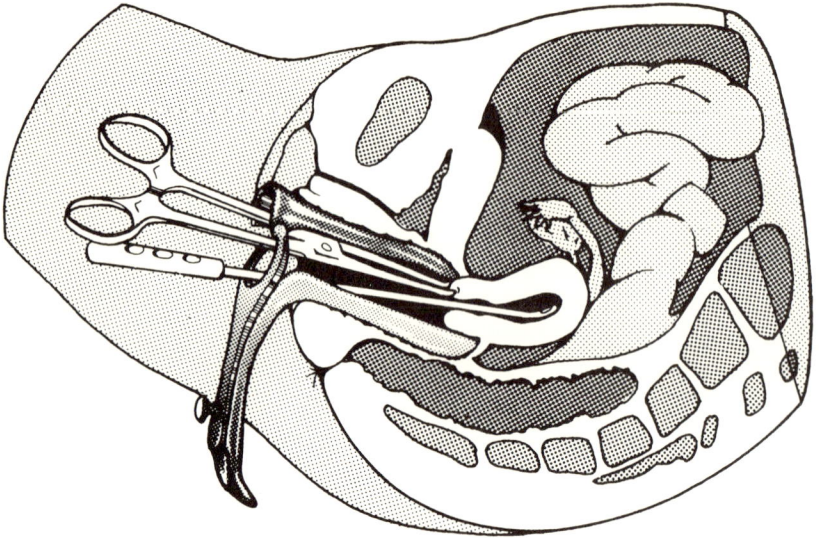

Figure 5.2 *Endometrial biopsy. A small piece of tisue is scraped from the lining of the uterus, removed, and sent for microscopic evaluation.*

physician grasps the cervix with a clamp to stabilize the uterus for the biopsy itself. The application of the clamp is associated with a sudden, sharp pinching sensation lasting for several seconds and usually well tolerated because the discomfort is so brief. Next, a thin metal tube, called a *curette*, is inserted through the cervix into the uterine cavity. The curette is then quickly withdrawn, scraping off a piece of the lining of the uterus. As the instrument is withdrawn the woman feels a cramp like a strong menstrual cramp. The discomfort lasts for about one minute and then dissipates over the next two to three minutes. The patient may experience some vaginal staining for up to several days following the biopsy. For this she may use a sanitary napkin or a

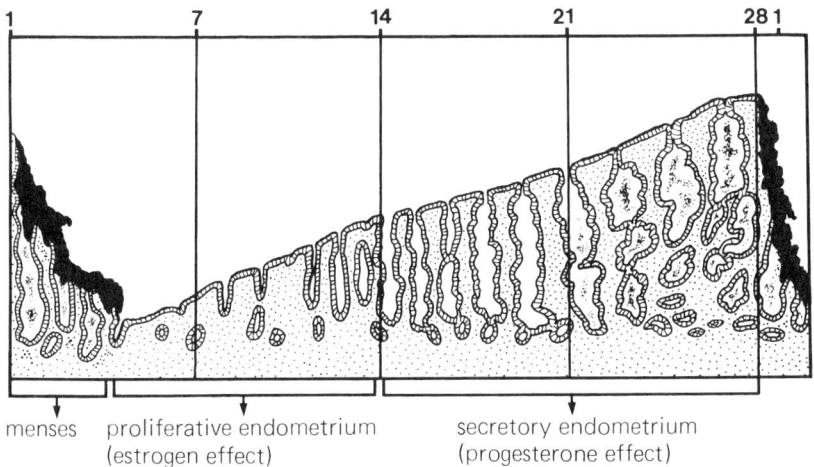

menses proliferative endometrium secretory endometrium
(estrogen effect) (progesterone effect)

Figure 5.3 *The lining of the uterus. The endometrium, the tissue lining the uterus, has one structure before ovulation (proliferative endometrium) and a different structure after ovulation (secretory endometrium). The secretory endometrium is a result of progesterone action in the endometrium. Since progesterone is only produced after ovulation, the presence of secretory endometrium is presumptive evidence that ovulation has occurred.*

tampon, whichever she usually uses for her menses. (See Figures 5.2 and 5.3.)

If the pathologist's report returns showing that ovulation did not occur and the temperature curve confirms this, the physician may begin to conclude that the female member of the couple has not ovulated at least that particular cycle. If the report comes back consistent with ovulation and ovulation has occurred at a time consistent with the basal body temperature curve, then we may assume that indeed an egg has been released.

It is also possible that the report may return consistent with ovulation but the date of ovulation differs radically from the time estimated by the basal body temperature curve. In this case, the physician may conclude that ovulation has occurred but the patient is producing a lower than normal amount of progesterone. The biopsy can also tell the physician whether or not a chronic infection of the uterine cavity, such as tuberculosis, might exist.

i. Advantage

The advantage of the endometrial biopsy is that it provides data that is much more reliable than the basal body temperature in terms of confirming or denying that ovulation occurs.

ii. Disadvantages

Its disadvantages are that it is somewhat uncomfortable, but should be easily tolerated in most cases. Furthermore, if the patient has become pregnant during that particular cycle, in taking the endometrial biopsy there is a small chance that pregnancy may be interrupted, causing a miscarriage.

Progesterone Blood Level

Another test for ovulation is to measure progesterone levels directly. This can be done simply by drawing blood from the patient's arm at a time of the woman's cycle when the progesterone levels should be highest.

i. Advantages

The advantages of this test are that it is less uncomfortable than an endometrial biopsy and still gives excellent information about whether or not ovulation has occurred. Furthermore, the test provides direct and accurate information about progesterone levels following ovulation. It appears to be the best way to diagnose a luteal

ii. Disadvantage

phase deficiency. The disadvantage is that the test provides no information about the normality or abnormality of the tissue lining the uterine cavity. Only an endometrial biopsy can provide this information. Many infertility specialists use both the endometrial biopsy and a plasma progesterone level done at the mid-luteal phase (about one week after

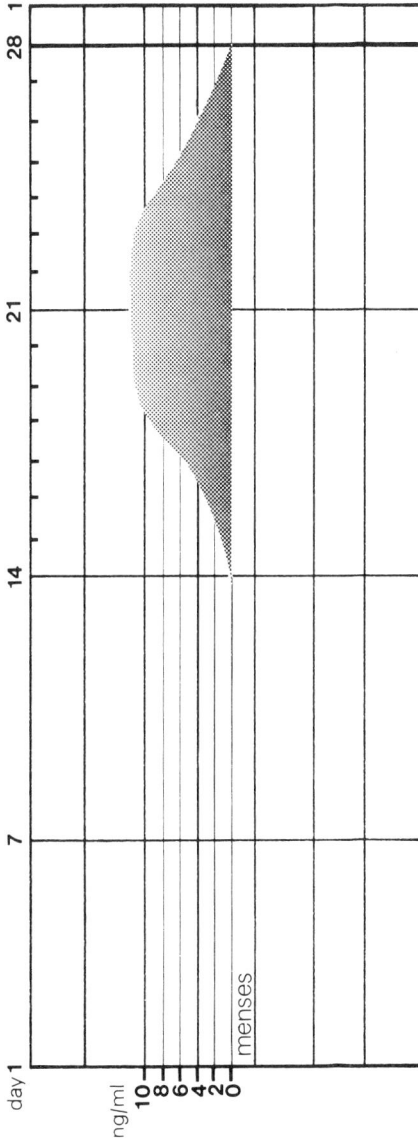

Figure 5.4 *Changes in plasma progesterone during the cycle. After ovulation the blood level of progesterone gradually increases, reaches its maximum between cycle days 20 and 23, and then gradually diminishes. Progesterone is produced only after ovulation. Thus, finding a significant blood level of this hormone is presumptive evidence of ovulation. This is best done between cycle days 19 and 24.*

the expected ovulation) to investigate ovulation. (See Figure 5.4.)

The third group of infertility tests are those that study the structure of the uterus and Fallopian tubes. It is impossible for a woman to achieve pregnancy by ordinary means without having at least one open tube through which an egg might be picked up and in which fertilization of that ovum can take place. Repeated loss of pregnancy may occur if the uterine cavity is distorted or abnormal in shape. If the uterine cavity is so distorted that most of the cavity is absent, pregnancy may never occur at all. Thus, evaluation of the uterine cavity and both Fallopian tubes is very important. This aspect of fertility may be evaluated indirectly through the *Rubin's Insufflation test*, more directly by a specialized x-ray procedure called a *hysterosalpingogram*, or most directly and accurately by *endoscopy*. Endoscopy is a technique of directly examining the structure and working of the human body by inserting a small telescope into different parts of the body. The three types of endoscopy, hysteroscopy, culdoscopy and laparoscopy will be discussed later in this chapter.

Rubin's Insufflation Test

The principle behind the Rubin's Insufflation test is simple. If one were to take a certain amount of gas and use it to inflate a balloon, as the balloon expands the pressure inside will build up. If a machine that will draw a graph of the increasing pressure were attached to the balloon, one would get a curve of a certain shape. If the same balloon had two holes in it and the same amount of gas were pumped into it, the pressure produced in the balloon would be less. As the gas was pumped in at one end some of it would leak out of the balloon through the two holes. The curve made by the machine would be of different shape than when the balloon had no holes. This is precisely the principle of the Rubin's test. A pressure tube, connected to a machine which records pressure, is connected to the cervix and carbon dioxide gas is allowed to slowly enter the uterine cavity. If the woman has two open Fallopian tubes present, (i.e., the channel within the tube is not blocked), as the gas flows into the uterine cavity some of it will leak out through the tubes. The gas will flow out into the abdominal cavity and irritate the patient's diaphragm. Strangely enough, when the diaphragm is irritated the patient does not feel abdominal pain but shoulder pain. The result is that if carbon dioxide gas leaks out of the uterine cavity through open Fallopian tubes, the patient will feel shoulder pain. As the machine records the pressure in the uterine cavity a curve is drawn and it is noted that the pressure within the uterine cavity does not rise as rapidly as it would if none of the gas had leaked out. If the patient, on the other hand, had both tubes closed by previous surgery or resulting from a previous inflammatory process, then the carbon dioxide placed within the uterine cavity would not leak out. The patient would feel no shoulder pain and the pressure within the uterine cavity would build up very, very rapidly. The result would be a graph with a characteristic shape.

The advantages of the Rubin's test is that it can *i. Advantages* be done in the physician's office with a limited amount of apparatus other than the Rubin's insufflation machine. No exposure to x-rays is required. The disadvantages are that the information is not terribly accurate. The Rubin's test offers general information as to whether there is at least one Fallopian tube open or closed. It cannot tell the physician anything about the shape of the uterine cavity, whether or not one tube is open and the other closed, or both tubes partially open. If both tubes are closed, the test offers no information as to where in the Fallopian tube the point of obstruction exists. If the test is normal, a hysterosalpingogram is still done to investigate the contour of the uterine cavity and to rule out the possiblity of adhesions about the outside of the Fallopian tube. If the test is abnormal, indicating a possible obstruction of the Fallopian tube, the x-ray is still done to confirm the findings of the Rubin's test and to help locate the portion of the Fallopian tube in which the obstruction exists. Because both a normal and an abnormal finding of the Rubin's test still necessitates the use of a *hysterosalpingogram* for further information, many physicians have stopped using the Rubin's test.

Hysterosalpingo-gram

The word hysterosalpingogram is so long and complicated in sound that it frequently makes people run and hide. The very sound of the word conjures up visions of a grotesque procedure that was designed to test the limits of human endurance. But, like so many words in medicine, the term hysterosalpingogram is composed of smaller words that describe exactly what the procedure is designed to do. *Hystero* refers to the uterus. *Salpingo* refers to the Fallopian tubes. The *gram* part of it describes a picture. The result is a word meaning a "picture of the uterus and tubes" which is exactly what one desires when one is evaluating a woman for infertility. In this procedure the woman is taken into a radiologist's suite and is asked to lie upon an x-ray table. A tube with a rubber gasket is inserted into the cervix and into the uterine cavity. The tube is

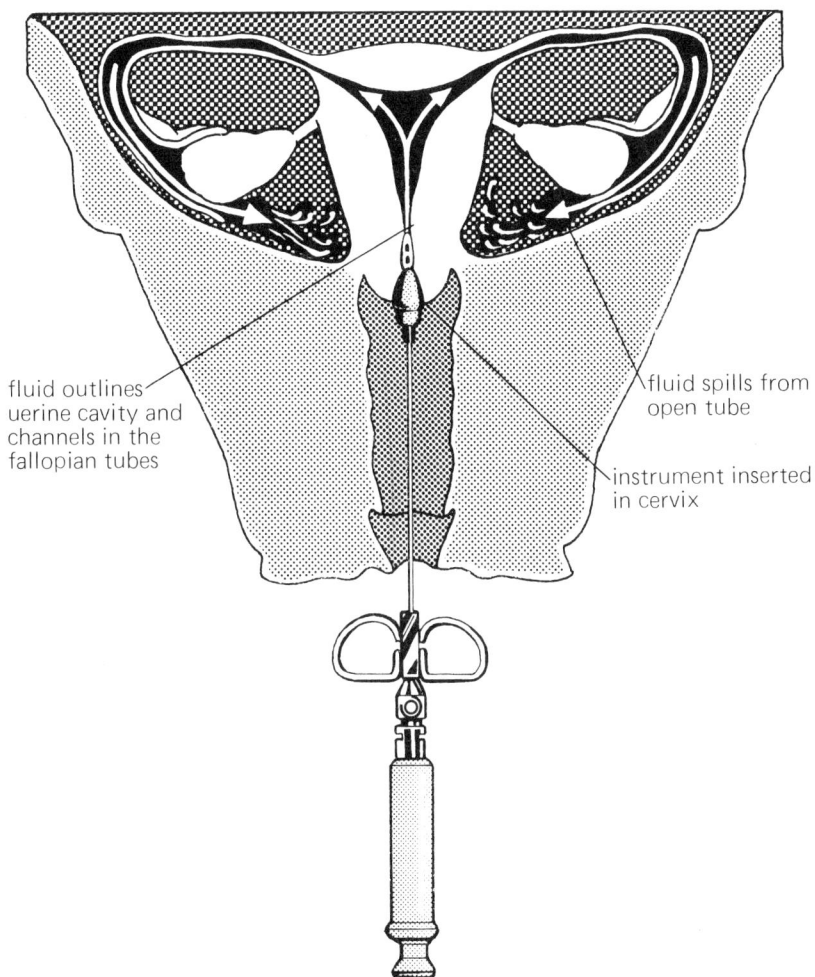

fluid outlines
uerine cavity and
channels in the
fallopian tubes

fluid spills from
open tube

instrument inserted
in cervix

Figure 5.5 *Hysterosalpinogram. By injecting a fluid which can be seen on x-ray, one is able to take pictures of the cavity of the uterus and the tubes.*

connected to a syringe containing a fluid that can be seen on x-ray. An x-ray can show bony structures but soft, muscular structures such as the uterus and tubes will not show up on a conventional x-ray film. By gently pushing the plunger down on the syringe the contrast fluid goes through the metal tube into the uterine cavity. By taking x-rays at this time the physician can see the outline of the contrast material which has filled the cavity. The result is a silhouette of the uterine cavity. As the dye completely fills the uterine cavity, it begins to pour out through the Fallopian tubes, filling the channels in the tubes and eventually pouring out the ends of the tubes. If there is an obstruction in the tube the dye will stop at that point. The result is that one is able to locate the point of obstruction if it exists. If there is something projecting into the uterine cavity such as a fibroid, (a benign tumor), or extending into the uterine cavity such as a septum, a fibroid on a stalk or a polyp, these defects will be visualized on x-ray. As you can see, the hysterosalpingogram is a very helpful procedure and, short of endoscopy, which will be discussed below, provides the maximum amount of information about the internal structure of the female reproductive system. (See Figures 5.5, 5.6, 5.7, 5.8, and 5.9.)

As the fluid fills the uterine cavity during a hysterosalpingogram, the uterus becomes slightly stretched and the patient may feel some discomfort. The sensation is usually described as feeling like a moderate menstrual cramp and lasts for about two to three minutes longer than the actual injecting of fluid. The whole period of discomfort lasts for about ten minutes and is easily tolerated by most patients.

i. Advantage   The advantages of the hysterosalpingogram are

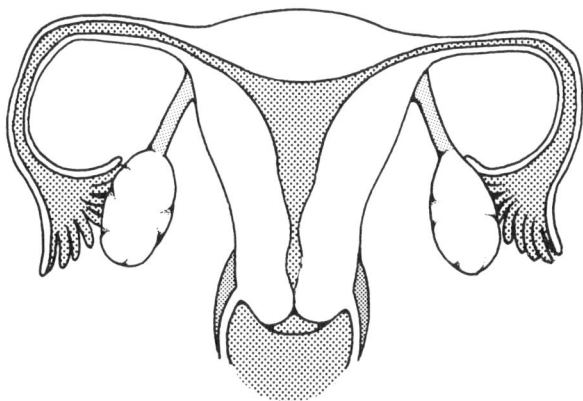

anatomy

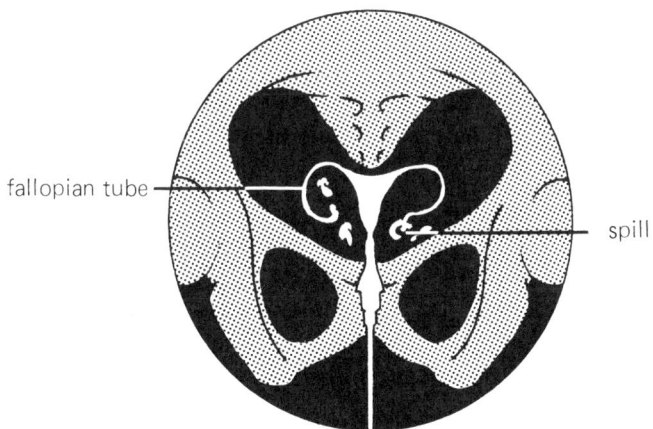

fallopian tube

spill

x-ray

Figure 5.6 *Normal hysterosalpingogram*

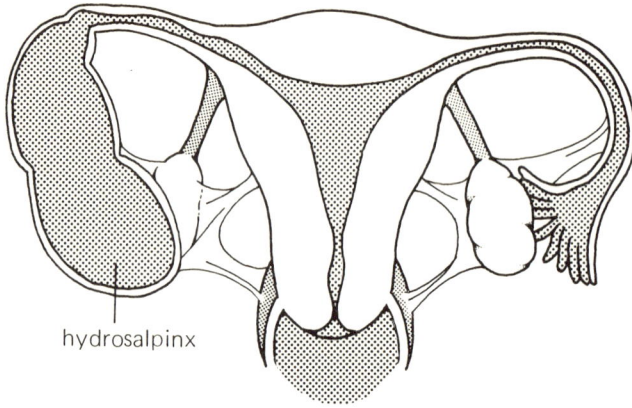

anatomy

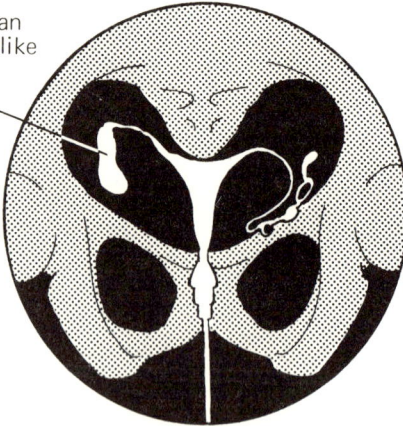

hydrosalpinx—an obstructed sac-like tube

x-ray

Figure 5.7 *Hysterosalpingogram showing closure of one tube.*

fibroid

anatomy

fibroid outlined on hysterosalpingogram

x-ray

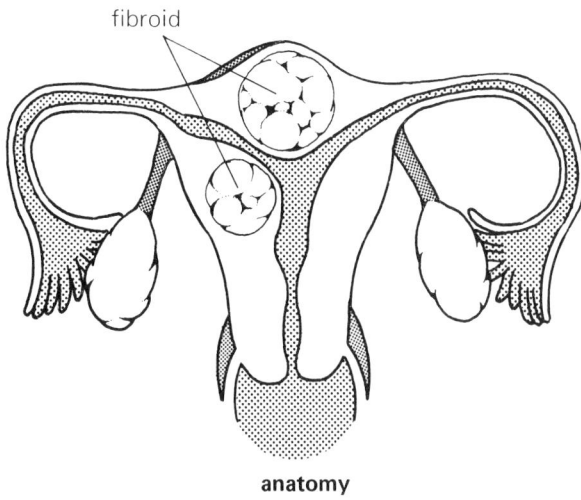

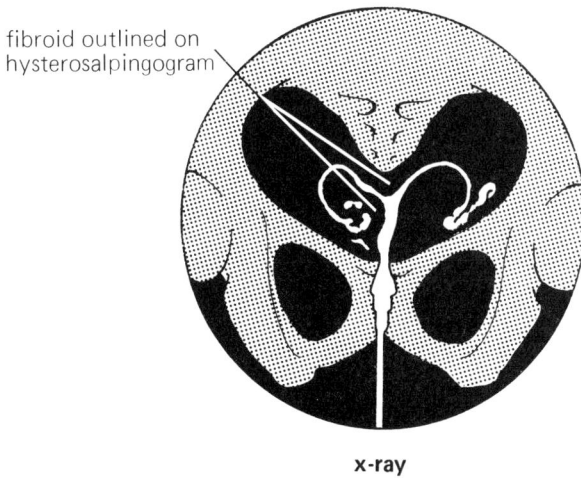

Figure 5.8 *Hysterosalpingogram showing distortion of the cavity of the uterus by fibroids.*

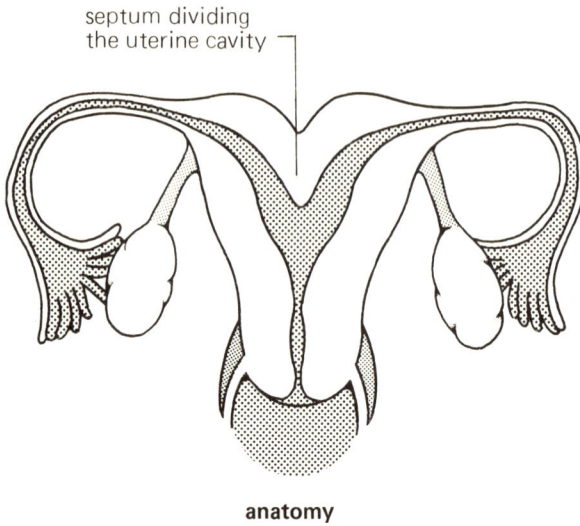

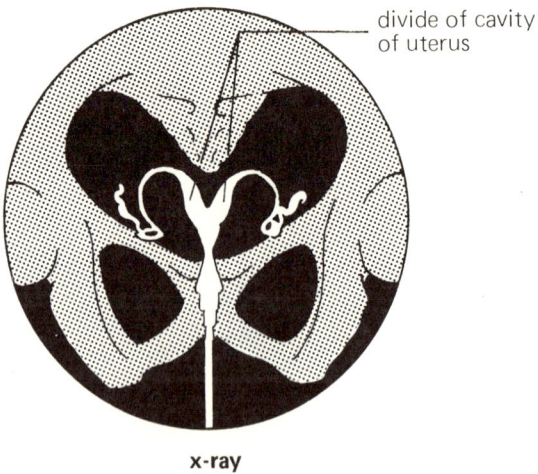

Figure 5.9 *Hysterosalpingogram showing the upper portion of the cavity of the uterus divided by a septum (wall).*

that it provides the maximum amount of information about the female reproductive system short of utilizing endoscopy. Like all things, the hysterosalpingogram has its disadvantages. Firstly, it is an x-ray procedure. As an x-ray procedure it involves subjecting the patient to radiation. The dose of radiation is small and therefore the risk to the patient is not great. The hysterosalpingogram is scheduled during the first half of the woman's cycle. The reason for this is that it is performed prior to ovulation to prevent the possibility of irradiating a fertilized egg. The second disadvantage is that it is not 100% accurate. However, it is significantly more accurate in its positive and negative findings than the Rubin's test. Nevertheless, it is still only 70% accurate. This means that a certain number of times the x-ray will show that there is something wrong in either the uterine cavity or the tube when in fact there will be nothing wrong at all. Conversely, there will be times when there is, in fact, something wrong with either the uterus or the Fallopian tubes and the x-ray will be apparently normal. The most common reason for this is that the x-ray, by photographing the contrast fluid within the uterine cavity and the channels within the Fallopian tubes, shows the cavities within the organs rather than the tissues of which the organ is made. It fails to show its outside surfaces. It is possible for adhesions to be on the outside of the Fallopian tube distorting the tube and holding it in such a position that pickup of a released egg is impossible. Since the channel of the tube may be open and normal, the x-ray will appear to be normal, giving no hint of the adhesions on the outside. The result is that findings of the hysterosal-

ii. Disadvantages

pingogram should be confirmed by endoscopy.

Endoscopy is placing a telescope-like device into a portion of the body and looking through it to view that particular organ directly with the eye, without the aid of x-ray or any other indirect means. Generally, it is one of the most accurate diagnostic procedures available. There are three forms of endoscopy that are relevant to infertility. These are hysteroscopy, culdoscopy and laparoscopy. *Hysteroscopy* is a means of looking at the contents of the uterine cavity directly. *Culdoscopy* and *laparoscopy* are ways of looking at the outside surface of the uterus and Fallopian tubes to evaluate their function and condition by direct visualization.

Hysteroscopy

For hysteroscopy, a patient lies down on her back, and under local or general anesthesia, the opening of the uterus, the cervix, is slightly stretched. An instrument is then inserted through the opening of the cervical canal and the cavity of the uterus is inflated with either carbon dioxide gas or a clear fluid. When the cavity is distended so that the front and back walls of the cavity are no longer touching, a telescope-like device is inserted through the cervix into the uterine cavity. The physician then can look around and study the surfaces of the uterine cavity. The area where the Fallopian tubes join the uterus can be visualized from the inside and the actual opening of the tube on the inside of the uterus can be studied. Polyps, fibroids on stalks, and various other structures projecting into the uterine cavity that should not normally be present may be removed under direct visualization using special instruments and the hysteroscope. The presence of a septum (wall) projecting into the uterine cavity can be confirmed and under certain

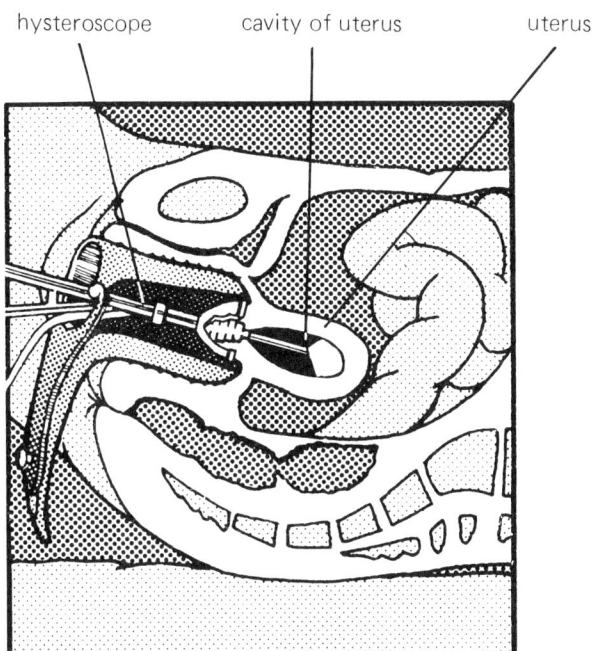

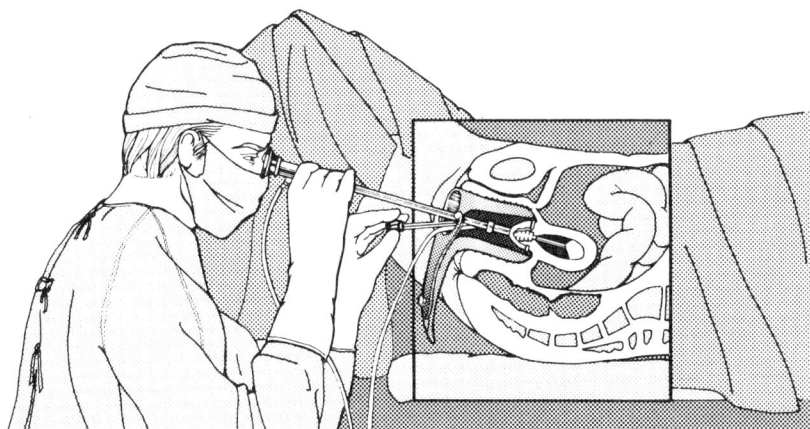

Figure 5.10 *Hysteroscopy. By inserting the hysteroscope into the vagina and through the cervix, the cavity of the uterus can be seen and evaluated.*

circumstances, the septum can actually be cut away under hysteroscopic control. Using the hysteroscope, adhesions within the uterine cavity that may abnormally hold the front and back walls of the cavity together, thereby partially obliterating the cavity, may be located and cut. (See Figure 5.10.)

i. Advantage

The advantage of hysteroscopy is that it allows direct visualization of the contents of the uterine cavity. Under certain circumstances, a diagnosis made by a hysterosalpingogram can be confirmed by hysteroscopy and treatment may be accomplished using the hysteroscope. Cutting an intrauterine adhesion or the removal of an intrauterine polyp or a lost IUD are examples of its most common uses. Treatment can be done under direct visualization rather than using a blind procedure such as a dilatation and curettage. Most other endoscopic procedures associated with infertility are done under general anesthesia or very deep sedation. Hysteroscopy is most frequently done under general anesthesia but under appropriate circumstances, may be done only under local anesthesia, thereby minimizing the risk to the patient. There are really very few risks with hysteroscopy.

There are times when it is very helpful to look at the Fallopian tubes directly. The methods described thus far of determining whether or not a woman's tubes are open, do not provide any detailed information about the outside of the Fallopian tubes and may be associated with a significant degree of error. In an attempt to seek more precise information, an effort to actually look at the Fallopian tube in the patient has been made. For this, a telescope is inserted into the abdomen and aimed toward the uterus, Fallopian tubes and ovaries. The uterus is filled with a dye solution in much the same way as it was for a hysterosalpingogram and using the endoscope, the dye solution can be observed to fill and spill out of the Fallopian tubes. This will confirm the degree to which the tubes are open or closed. Since the outside surface of the tubes may be seen, any possible adhesions that are present may be visualized. Under certain circumstances, additional instruments may be inserted and, if the adhesions are in the proper place, they may be cut. Other pathology may be observed such as abnormalities of the ovaries or abnormalities of the tubes. These may not be correctable using endoscopic instruments and the need for regular abdominal surgery may be decided upon.

For the insertion of the endoscope one of two *Laparoscopy* routes may be selected. The route chosen determines the kind of instrument used. Today, the most common route is through the umbilicus or belly-button, hence, the everyday term "belly-button surgery." Here, the woman is placed on an operating table, lying on her back and is usually given general anesthesia. It should be noted that under certain circumstances, local anesthesia has been used. A small incision is made in the lower edge of the umbilicus and the abdomen is then inflated with carbon dioxide gas. A telescope-like device, called a *laparoscope* is inserted through the same incision in the umbilicus and as just described, the abdominal and pelvic contents are visualized and studied. (See Figure 5.11.)

Another route involves the back wall of the *Culdoscopy* vagina. As the illustration shows, by making a hole

119

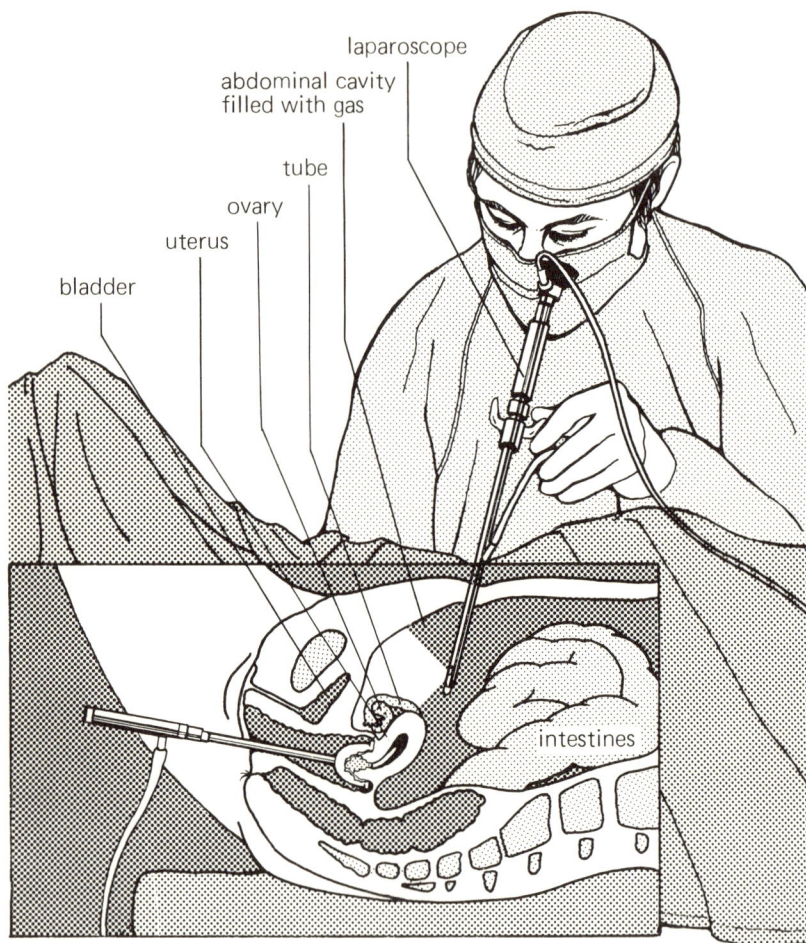

Figure 5.11 *Laparoscopy. By inserting the laparoscope through the navel of a patient, the physician can see and evaluate much of the contents of the abdomen, including the uterus, Fallopian tubes and ovaries.*

in the back wall of the vagina, just below the cervix, one can easily enter the abdominal cavity. By deeply sedating a patient, placing her on an operating table with her chest down, and then bringing her knees toward her chest (this is sometimes called a "knee-chest position"), the vagina is directed back toward the surgeon. Instruments are inserted into the vagina to expose the back wall of the vagina and a small incision is made just above the cervix. Through this incision a telescope-like device is inserted, called a *culdoscope*. Using the culdoscope, the back surface of the uterus, the Fallopian tubes and ovaries may be studied in the same way as under laparoscopy. Dye may be seen filling and spilling out of both tubes. Adhesions may be located and with instruments inserted next to the culdoscope, the adhesions may be cut and other limited surgical procedures accomplished. The need for further surgery may be ascertained during culdoscopy. (See Figure 5.12.)

The advantages of both procedures are that they allow accurate information about the Fallopian tubes and the presence or absence of adhesions about them that is not available through any other means. Therefore, whenever Fallopian tube functioning is considered as a possible reason for infertility, culdoscopy or laparoscopy should be a necessary procedure in the patient's evaluation. *i. Advantages*

The risks versus the benefits of these procedures must be weighed by both the physician and the patient. The risks of either of these procedures are the normal risks of abdominal surgery. They include the possibility of damage to any of the abdominal organs. In the hands of an experienced physician the risks are minimal and the benefits, in *ii. Disadvantages*

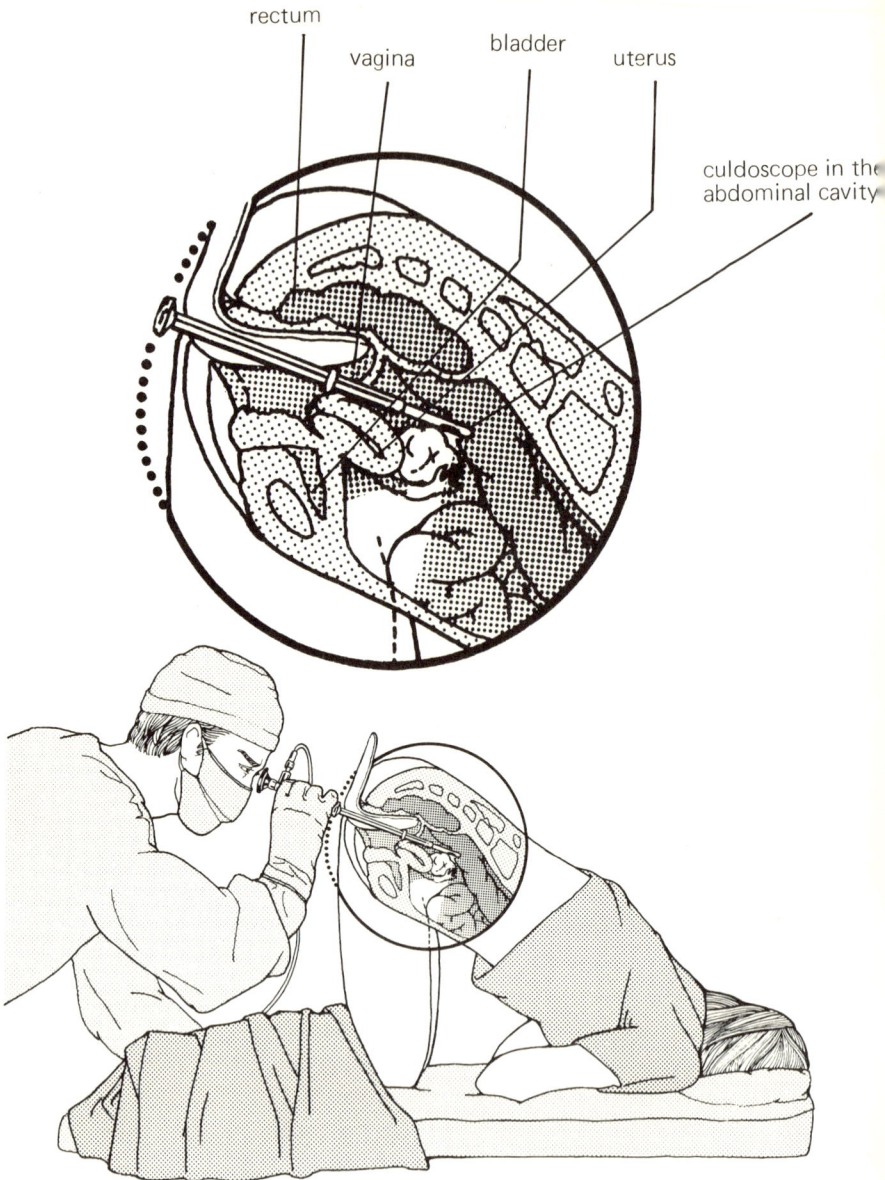

rectum

vagina

bladder

uterus

culdoscope in the abdominal cavity

Figure 5.12 *Culdoscopy. By inserting the culdoscope through the back of the vagina, the physician can see and evaluate the ovaries, Fallopian tubes and the back of the uterus.*

122

terms of information gained and possible treatment, are enormous.

The fourth category of infertility testing involves the interaction of the male sperm and seminal fluid and the female genital tract. One wishes to test the survival of the sperm within the reproductive tract of the female partner. The *post-coital test*, sometimes called the *Simms-Huhner test*, is the most common means of testing this component of reproduction. In this test, the man and woman are asked to have intercourse at mid-cycle and are seen several hours later at the physician's office. The woman is then examined in very much the same kind of position as she would be for a routine Pap smear. The physician, using a long, thin tube like a straw, attached to a syringe, sucks off some of the secretion from within the genital tract. The usual technique involves taking some of the fluid from within the vagina and taking separate specimens from three points progressively further up the canal within the cervix. Each specimen is put on a separate slide and studied under the microscope. The examining physician is looking for live sperm cells in each specimen. Finding live sperm cells indicates that, at least grossly, the male and female are having intercourse properly and that the sperm is surviving within the woman.

It must be emphasized that in looking for a reason for infertility, nothing must be taken for granted. The possiblity that the couple does not know how to have sexual relations must always be entertained. If the semen analysis demonstrates the presence of live sperm and the post-coital examination fails to show any sperm within the vagina, then regardless of what the couple has told the physician,

Male-Female Interaction (Fourth Basic Group of Tests)

Post-coital Test

the evidence indicates that the man is not delivering sperm into the woman's vagina. The possibility of a problem with sexual technique must be strongly entertained. If the post-coital test indicates live sperm within the vagina and cervix, one knows that the couple has been using a technique that is good enough to allow the delivery of live sperm into the vagina. It is also possible to see live sperm in the vaginal specimen and non-moving sperm in the specimen taken from the cervix. This indicates that there is something within the female reproductive tract that is killing off the sperm placed there during intercourse. The possible explanations are several. There may be an allergic reaction where the woman's bodily defenses that would ordinarily kill off foreign micro-organisms may falsely identify the sperm cells as a foreign organism and kill them. Another possibility is an infection of the female reproductive tract with a micro-organism that provides a hostile environment for the sperm and causes the death of the sperm.

In the above descriptions it is assumed that there is a large quantity of watery, clear mucus present within the cervix to support the life of the sperm cells for the test. Since this test is being done at mid-cycle, at the time that ovulation should occur, this would indicate that there should be cervical mucus present to act as a medium through which the sperm cells can swim on their way up through the cervix to the uterus, the Fallopian tube to the egg. It is possible for the woman to make a very small amount of cervical mucus or to make a cervical mucus that is so thick that instead of acting as a pathway for the sperm on its way up to the egg, the cervical mucus acts as a barrier. The examining

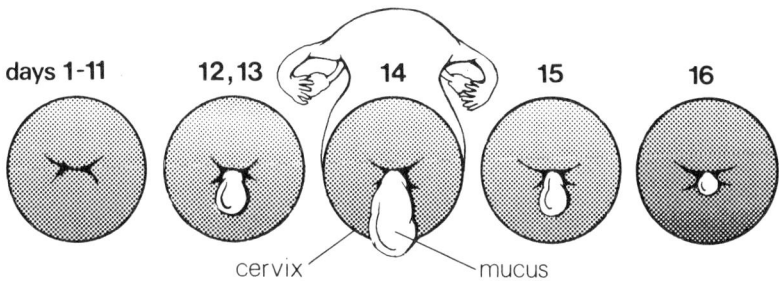

Figure 5.13 *Cervical mucus. At the time of ovulation, the mucus produced by the cervix changes in volume and quantity. Before and after ovulation, there is a small amount of very thick viscous mucus present. At ovulation and a day or so before and after, the volume of mucus increases and the quality changes to a clear watery liquid. Finding a large volume of clear watery cervical mucus is presumptive evidence of ovulation on or around the day of examination. Since such mucus allows sperm to enter the uterus and survive for a longer period, ovulation time is the best time to perform a post-coital test.*

physician then sees on post-coital examination, some live sperm in the vagina, a small or moderate amount of cervical mucus within the cervix which is so thick that it is very difficult to suck it up for microscopic study. When the specimen is finally put on the slide and studied under the microscope, few, if any sperm cells are seen. If any are seen they are noted to be trapped in the mucus, unable to move forward or back or to progress from side to side. (See Figure 5.13.)

The advantages of the post-coital test are that it is a relatively simple test to do and can give a great deal of information. It can tell the physician about the cervical mucus production of the woman, the survival of the sperm within the female reproductive tract and can also give the physician a general idea of the quality of sperm production of the male

i. Advantages

125

partner. It involves no risk to either member of the couple.

Immunological or Antibody Testing   If the cervical mucus production is good but the survival of the sperm cells within the cervical mucus is poor, then further testing is indicated. In most cases, the possibility of an immunological problem must be considered. Both the male and the female should be studied for antisperm antibodies.

As outlined above, another possible explanation for poor sperm survival with an adequate cervical mucus could be an infection of the reproductive tract by a micro-organism. Cultures of both the male and the female reproductive tract for T-strain mycoplasma should be considered. This remains a controversial area of study.

If all of the basic studies outlined thus far have failed to demonstrate any reason for the couple's inability to have achieved a pregnancy, immunological studies of both members of the couple should still be performed. There is a certain incidence of antisperm antibodies in either the male or the female even in the face of a normal post-coital test. Though this is fairly uncommon a situation, it must be considered when no other reason for infertility can be found.

One performs tests, presumably, to find answers to questions. We hope to find why a man and woman have been unable to produce a child. It is surprising that sometimes tests may end up asking more questions rather than providing a definite answer. When one finds that ovulation is not occurring as determined by basal body temperature, endometrial biopsy, and/or plasma progesterone levels, one must then ask why? When one finds that sperm is not surviving within the female

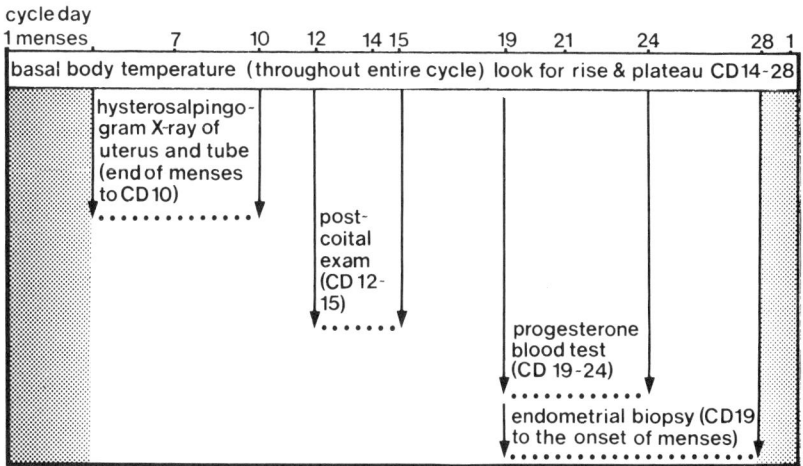

Figure 5.14 *Timing of infertility tests.*
A. *Basal body temperature. This should be taken throughout the cycle. A sustained elevation in the curve in the second half of the cycle is consistent with ovulation.*

B. *Hysterosalpingogram. This x-ray of the uterus and tubes should be taken after the end of menses and before the time of ovulation. To be sure to avoid ovulation one frequently selects cycle day 10 or 11 as the last day for taking the x-ray.*

C. *Post-coital examination. This test is to evaluate how well sperm lives in the cervical mucus of the woman being evaluated. The cervical mucus produced at the time of ovulation is best able to support the life of sperm. For this reason this test is usually scheduled between cycle days 12 and 15 of a 28-day cycle.*

D. *Progesterone blood test. Plasma progesterone is measured in a sample of blood drawn around the time of greatest progesterone production. This test is done between cycle days 19 and 24.*

E. *Endometrial biopsy. A sample of the tissue lining the uterus is removed and studied microscopically. If the sample was removed after ovulation, the tissue should have the structure of secretory endometrium. This tissue is best developed after cycle day 18. Thus, the biopsy or sampling of the endometrium is usually done between cycle day 19 and the onset of menses.*

127

reproductive tract, one must then ask why, because the answer to this question determines how easily the problem can be treated. If the woman has an obstruction of a Fallopian tube, one must ask where is that obstruction and how extensive is it because the probability of surgical success hinges on the answer.

Though a physician may lay out a plan of several tests at the initial consultation, other tests may prove necessary during the course of the workup. The trip from beginning to end may be long and at times seem complicated, but if you know why and how each test is done, the trip seems less involved and is easier to make. Make your physician your partner in this trip. Share your feelings and your fears with him. Try to understand his reasoning and his conclusions at each point in the investigation. These tests are to be done for you and not to you. All three people, the man and the woman of the couple, and the physician consulted, must take equal involvement.

Now that we have discussed the tests to be performed, let us progress to the treatment available.

Chapter 6

Infertility Therapy

THUS FAR, THE NORMAL PRODUCTION of a child has been discussed. Following this, the various steps that might break down resulting in infertility were outlined. Thus, it became clear that infertility, rather than being a specific disease, is a symptom. The next step was to discuss the various diagnostic techniques available to help pinpoint what the cause or causes of the inability to conceive might be. The purpose of this chapter is to present the treatments available to correct the specific problems found.

This entire chapter may easily be summarized by saying that therapy in each case must be applied to correct whatever abnormalities were found in the infertility investigation. If a structural problem was found then the structure of the reproductive system must somehow be returned to normal. If a hormonal problem existed then that must be corrected.

Prior to beginning therapy, a complete infertility evaluation must be completed. This evaluation cannot stop when one specific reason for infertility is found. It is possible that in a given couple more than one cause for infertility may exist. It would be unfortunate if treatment were started after finding a single problem and, after six months or a year of unsuccessful therapy, the infertility evaluation were completed only to find that there was a second problem that was never even suspected. Infertility is a problem of couples, not of individuals and the probability of success in the treatment of infertility is the total success possible after evaluation and treatment of both members of the couple.

I
MALE

The first step in the evaluation of the male member of the couple is a semen analysis. If it is not normal, even after a second analysis for confirmation, a physical examination and laboratory studies are ordered. X-ray studies and a testicular biopsy may be considered in some cases, as discussed in Chapter 5.

Medical
Treatment

If the studies have revealed that a hormonal problem exists, treatment must be directed toward the replacement or correction of the particular problem discovered. If the man has a pituitary malfunction resulting in low levels of the pituitary hormones FSH and LH, then the patient should be given FSH and LH. FSH is usually give in the form of *Human Menopausal Gonadotropin*, marketed under the name of *Pergonal*. Pergonal is a white powder which is dissolved in saline and administered by injection. Though it contains both FSH and LH, frequently additional LH stimulus is given in the form of injections of *HCG* or *Human Chorionic Gonadotropin*. HCG is also a white powder that is dissolved in saline and administered by injection. If thyroid problems are noted then one of various forms of thyroid hormones may be administered to replace those that are missing. Similarly, the adrenal glands that are not functioning up to normal activity may be supplemented by corticosteroids administered by mouth. The basic concept of returning to the body what the body is not producing is adhered to.

It should be noted that thyroid or corticosteroid medication should only be given after laboratory tests show a deficient function of the appropriate gland. In the past, these drugs had been given even in the face of a normally functioning adrenal or thyroid. The benefit to a man or woman with a normal thyroid or adrenal gland who is nonetheless given thyroid or corticosteroids must be questioned.

A great deal of attention and frustration has been directed toward the male who has a poor sperm count but who has a normal physical examination and laboratory studies. A number of forms of therapy have been tried. One of the older forms of treatment has been the use of corticosteroids or thyroid medication. As mentioned above, little or no success has been demonstrated with the use of such medication in the face of normal functioning of these endocrine organs. The use of testosterone, to suppress sperm production in the hope that when the medication is stopped, sperm production will rebound to higher levels, has also been tried. This form of therapy is known as *testosterone rebound therapy*, and it too has been questioned in recent years. Indeed, its potential for harm by suppressing sperm count and its failure to return even to pre-treatment levels is a hazard. Recently, various regimens using Clomiphene Citrate, Human Chorionic Gonadotropin (HCG), and/or Pergonal (HMG), have been tried. Though the use of these drugs must be considered experimental at this point, its potential for success in selected cases of the so-called "normal infertile males" is very promising.

In men who have an obstruction of the vas deferens that has been demonstrated using x-ray procedures, microsurgical techniques are now available to correct this problem. Here the blocked segment of the vas deferens is excised (cut out) and the cut segments anastomosed (re-connected) under a microscope thus re-establishing continuity of the pathway for sperm release. Using microsurgical techniques approximately 60–80% of males will produce viable sperm in their ejaculates. Unfortunately, the pregnancy rate at this time appears to be only 35%. This may indicate an effect of male antisperm antibodies produced during the period of time that the vas deferens was obstructed in sperm collected within the testes.

Besides using microsurgical anastomosis of the vas deferens to correct a spontaneous obstruction of the vas deferens as described above, it is also currently being used for the reversal of previous vasectomy procedures which were done for male sterilization. The desire for the reversal of steriliza-tion has increased with the increased use of steriliza-tion procedures in general. Microsurgery is probably the best hope at this point for the return of fertility in those males and females who have undergone these procedures.

II
FEMALE
Hormonal
Replacement
Adrenal
Thyroid

Basic infertility evaluation of the female began with the studies of thyroid and adrenal function. If over- or under-activity of these glands is found, returning function to normal levels is an important first step in treatment. In the process of evaluating infertility in the female member of the couple, the woman may have been found to have a progesterone deficiency. This evaluation is made by drawing a blood sample in the middle of the second half of her cycle, at a time when progesterone levels should be at their highest (usually cycle day 20–24). If the progesterone is lower than expected, then the diagnosis of a progesterone deficiency is made. The woman can be treated either with progesterone replacement, or with Clomiphene Citrate. In the first case, progesterone replacement, progesterone can be given to a woman from an outside source rather than getting it from the corpus luteum of the ovary as would normally be the case. Progesterone can be given to the patient by injection or by vaginal suppositories. Another alternative the physician may select is to give the patient a drug called *Delalutin*. This drug is one of the natural chemical products of progesterone and administered by injection. The role of Clomiphene Citrate for the treatment of a progesterone deficiency will be discussed a bit later in this chapter.

Progesterone

Injection

Suppository

Delalutin

Clomiphene

If infertility studies have shown that a woman is not ovulating at all or is ovulating very rarely, the patient should be given drugs to induce regular ovulation. The most common drugs used to produce ovulation are Clomiphene Citrate (marketed under the name Clomid), Human Menopausal Gonodotropin (referred to as HMG and marketed as Pergonal) and Human Chorionic Gonadotropin (referred to as HCG and marketed as Pregnyl).

Producing Ovulation

Clomiphene Citrate was originally discovered when pharmaceutical companies were attempting to chemically construct new estrogens for use in oral contraceptives. One molecule produced was found to have very poor estrogen properties. However, it was noted by accident, to induce ovulation in women who previously had not ovulated.

Clomiphene

This drug was called Clomiphene Citrate. Clomiphene works by causing the ovulatory center in the hypothalamus to be stimulated. This, in turn,

Use in Anovulation stimulates the pituitary gland to release more FSH and LH. These hormones will act upon the ovary to cause a follicle to ripen, and eventually rupture, releasing an egg. The result is ovulation. Clomiphene, a tablet, is usually given in five day courses. The patient usually takes one or more tablets a day for five days. After several days ovulation occurs.

When one mentions the use of a fertility drug, many people immediately think of the newspaper stories describing the mixed feelings of an infertility couple who have been treated with a "fertility drug" and are now blessed with a "litter" of children. The drug referred to in the newspaper articles is usually Pergonal and not Clomiphene Citrate. Though Clomiphene may be associated with a slightly increased incidence of multiple births (twins, etc.), it must be realized that the vast majority of patients have one baby and that the multiple births are usually twins and not triplets, quadruplets or quintuplets. The use of Clomiphene Citrate is safer than the use of Pergonal. It is administered by mouth rather than by injection. The need for monitoring the patient who is taking the medication with daily laboratory studies does not exist with Clomiphene Citrate, as it does with Pergonal.

Clomiphene was originally produced to make estrogen. Indeed, its chemical structure is very similar to that of some currently used estrogens. Clomiphene diminishes the effect of estrogens already present in the body, and so it is called an "estrogen blocker" or an "anti-estrogen." The drug does this by occupying the sites on cell membranes usually filled by potent estrogens. When Clomiphene fills these sites it is as if no estrogen is there, and normal estrogenic effects do not occur. This mechanism acts on the hypothalamus causing it to stimulate the pituitary. The result is more FSH and LH produced and released from the pituitary. These hormones in turn stimulate the ovary and follicular development and ovulation follows.

The production of a large quantity of watery cervical mucus at the time of ovulation is dependent upon estrogenic stimulation. When Clomiphene is used, occasionally the estrogenic stimulus for this cervical mucus production is diminished resulting in very little cervical mucus production. With a small amount of cervical mucus production, it becomes difficult for the sperm to enter the uterus and find its way up to the tube and the egg. The result is a paradoxical one. A woman who is not ovulating, but has been able to produce cervical mucus, is given Clomiphene so that she will make and release eggs on a regular basis. The treatment may be successful in that she will ovulate every cycle, but now, she may not become pregnant because she is producing a small amount of thick cervical mucus. In essence, one problem, not ovulating, has been replaced by another, poor cervical mucus. Thus, it is important for the physician to do a post-coital test so that cervical mucus and the ability of sperm to survive in the mucus can be examined after the appropriate dose of Clomiphene has been determined. If cervical mucus production has been found to be reduced following Clomiphene therapy, a small amount of estrogen can be given concurrently to improve mucus quality and volume and to facilitate pregnancy.

*Use to Control
Time of Ovulation*

Clomiphene is also used to treat patients who have problems other than anovulation (non-ovulating). In some cases a woman may ovulate but ovulate very irregularly. If it is important that the time of ovulation be known so that sexual activity can be planned more easily or that special procedures can be performed such as artificial insemination (to be discussed later in this chapter), then Clomiphene may be administered. In this case Clomiphene can be used to make an irregularly ovulating woman ovulate more regularly and at known times. The fertile period can be known in advance and if the couple's schedules are complex, their personal lives can be arranged so that they can be sure of making love during the woman's most fertile days.

*Use in
Progesterone
Deficiency*

Another use for Clomiphene is to treat a woman with a progesterone deficiency. As described in an earlier chapter, progesterone is produced by the ovary after ovulation by a structure called the corpus luteum. The corpus luteum can be thought of as a progesterone producing factory and is a structure that is left over from the follicle after the egg is released. The follicle produces the cells that are later used to generate progesterone which readies the lining of the uterus for implantation of the fertilized egg. When a lower than normal level of progesterone is made it is thought to be a result of poor functioning of the corpus luteum cells. Since the cells come from the follicle there are some researchers who feel that the defect lies not in the corpus luteum itself but in the follicle from which it comes. By giving the patient Clomiphene, the follicle is stimulated by FSH and LH from the pituitary producing a more ripened follicle and presumably a better corpus luteum. Indeed, giving Clomiphene in one of several regimens does result in higher levels of progesterone production by the corpus luteum. It must be emphasized that this is not the only therapy for a progesterone deficiency. Rather than treating the corpus luteum, one may elect to administer progesterone directly by injection or vaginal suppository or one of its metabolites such as 17-hydroxy progesterone in the form of injectable Delalutin.

In giving Clomiphene for anovulation the patient is frequently treated with progressively increasing doses of the drug until a level of therapy is reached that produces an apparently normal ovulation. The determination that normal ovulation has occurred is done by one or more of the following methods. The patient is asked to take a *basal body temperature.* Then the patient and the physician look for a classic, biphasic basal body temperature curve that is usually associated with normal ovulation. As described earlier, the basal body temperature curve is a rather crude test. There are some patients who ovulate normally, who are incapable of generating a classical biphasic curve. Thus, the basal body temperature curve may be thought of as confirmatory but not diagnostic of ovulation. In other words, if it shows ovulation and other tests concur, then the basal body temperature curve may be thought of as supporting evidence that ovulation did result from the preceding therapy. If, on the other hand, the basal body temperature curve does not show ovulation but other tests are consistent with ovulation, the temperature curve should be ignored. The other tests are plasma progesterone levels drawn at approximately the mid-portion of the second half of the cycles and/or an endometrial biopsy. The plasma progesterone level should show elevation of plasma progesterone to levels that are usually found with normal ovulation. If ovulation has indeed occurred, then an endometrial biopsy should show a secretory endometrium. The usual, maximum dose of Clomiphene is four tablets a day for five days. It must be emphasized that there are several different regimens involving Clomiphene use and that the maximum Clomiphene dose accepted may vary from physician to physician.

If Clomiphene therapy is successful, the woman being treated will ovulate the cycle during which the drug is taken. Since the drug is essentially out of the body within days of its last dose its effect is not felt beyond the cycle in which it is administered. Therefore, if pregnancy does not occur, Clomiphene must be repeated monthly to maintain regular ovulation. The main indication for the use of Clomiphene Citrate is to induce ovulation in a woman who desires pregnancy. It is not used to produce regular menstrual cycles in a woman who does not desire pregnancy. For the latter situation other drugs can be used. Just as with any medication, care must be taken not to give Clomiphene to a pregnant woman for fear of theoretically affecting the unborn fetus.

Clomiphene and HCG

Assuming that ovulation has not occurred with the maximum dose of Clomiphene, then an additional cycle at the same dose, with an injection of a hormone called Human Chorionic Gonadotropin (HCG) at cycle day fourteen, is added. A certain percentage of patients will ovulate following the HCG injection who did not ovulate on Clomiphene alone. Approximately 80% of patients who were treated with Clomiphene who had been anovulatory will ovulate following Clomiphene administration. Of those 80%, in a six month course of therapy, approximately 40–50% will become pregnant. Of those patients who do not become pregnant, an additional percentage will respond to Clomiphene plus HCG therapy. Approximately 15% of the patients who do not ovulate are now left. These patients must be considered as candidates for combined Clomiphene, HMG (Pergonal), HCG therapy.

Clomiphene HMG and HCG

This 15% represents that group of women whose pituitary gland fails to produce increased amounts of FSH and LH in response to Clomiphene therapy. The physician has tried stimulating the hypothalamus to make the pituitary produce more FSH and LH in an effort to produce the maturation of the follicle and the release of an egg from an ovary. Since the pituitary has been unable to do this an obvious solution is to take FSH and LH from another source and give it to the patient, thereby completely bypassing the pituitary as a source of ovarian stimulation. This is precisely what is done with the administration of HMG (Pergonal).

HMG (Pergonal) is an injectable drug that represents crystallized, purified extract of FSH and LH obtained from the urine of menopausal women. Women in their early menopause produce large amounts of FSH and LH which is usually excreted in the urine. It was suggested years ago that an economically feasible way of collecting FSH and LH would be to extract and purify these hormones from menopausal urine which is rich in FSH and LH. This is precisely what has been done. By dissolving the crystalline substance in a small amount of fluid and injecting it into a woman whose

HMG (Pergonal)

pituitary does not produce FSH and LH, her ovaries can be stimulated to respond as they would not have before. Since these hormones are being administered exogeneously (from a source outside the body) the control of follicular development is less precise than under normal circumstances. The result is that approximately 20% of pregnancies resulting from HMG therapy are multiple births. Patients being given HMG should be carefully monitored for clinical response and laboratory studies should be used to follow estrogen production. Using monitoring, the incidence of multiple births has been reduced as has the incidence of over-stimulation of the ovary. Overstimulation of the ovaries is a complex clinical picture, known as *hyper-stimulation syndrome*, which results in the ovaries enlarging from their usual olive size to the size of oranges, grapefruits, or larger. If the ovaries become too large, the patient must be hospitalized and observed for several days. The use of HMG must be taken quite seriously and requires both the art and the science of medicine for its administration.

There are some patients who respond to Clomiphene by producing a small amount of FSH and LH but not enough to stimulate the ovary to actual ovulation. These patients need not go to treatment with HMG alone, but can benefit by treatment with Clomiphene, HMG and HCG. The selection of which regimen, Clomiphene alone, Clomiphene and HMG and HCG, or HMG and HCG, must be left to the physician. Of the women treated with HMG over 95% will ovulate. Approximately 50% will become pregnant. The reason that not all of the women who ovulate become pregnant is that not infrequently more than one problem will exist. By inducing ovulation the other causes of infertility have not necessarily been corrected or are correctable.

A new drug, available in the United Kingdom, Canada, Europe, and in the United States, is *bromocryptine.* It induces ovulation in certain types of patients who may not respond to Clomiphene. Bromocryptine is used to treat patients who have a specific kind of endocrine problem — elevated blood levels of a hormone called *Prolactin.* These patients clinically have amenorrhea and a breast discharge. In a recent study, this drug has been found to be useful in treating ordinary patients who are anovulatory. A complete discussion of bromocryptine is beyond the scope of this book. At this point I just want to mention the existence of this new medication, that it can be given by mouth rather than injection and that it holds great promise for the near future in treating the infertile anovulatory woman.

Bromocryptine

In summary, if infertility is a result of a hormonal imbalance, whether of thyroid, adrenal or hypothalamic-pituitary origin, the female usually ovulates very few times or not at all during the course of a year. These patients are usually said to be *anovulatory.* Ovulation can usually be restored by treating the hormonal problem directly, by substituting the missing body substances.

In the event of a structural abnormality such as an abnormally shaped uterus or closed Fallopian tubes, no administration of medication can be of help. The only solution is a surgical restoration of anatomy. The diagnosis of such a problem has usually been made by hysterosalpingogram and

Structural Problems

141

confirmed by endoscopy, be it hysteroscopy, culdoscopy or laparoscopy. Once the problem has been defined a surgical approach must be considered.

In a woman, the structural abnormalities may be associated with the vagina, the cervix, the uterus or the Fallopian tubes. It is possible for the woman to have a long wall, running lengthwise down the vagina, acting as a partial obstruction to proper intercourse. Another possible obstruction of the vagina may be a wall extending from side-to-side, partially obstructing the vagina. This may be an unusually thick hymen or a wall further in within the vagina that effectively seals off the route through which sperm would enter the cervix. In each case the surgical solution is fairly simple. The wall (septum) is surgically removed and the continuity of the vagina is returned.

Vagina

Uterus

The uterus may have some structures distorting its cavity, projecting into the uterine cavity or somehow affecting the surface area of the cavity. This may be a result of a *fibroid*, technically known as a myoma, or a *septum* (wall), projecting into the uterine cavity. A fibroid is a benign tumor found in approximately 20% of all women. In many cases it may be present in various sizes and have absolutely no reproductive significance. However, if the mass is in such a position as to distort the uterine cavity or to partially close off one or both of the Fallopian tubes, surgical treatment should be considered. It may manifest itself by causing infertility, by preventing pregnancy, or by causing recurrent miscarriages (habitual abortions). In the latter case, pregnancy occurs but the growing embryo impinges upon the fibroid and is compromised by it, causing

Fibroid
Septum

disruption and death of the pregnancy. The diagnosis of the presence of a fibroid may be made by hysterosalpingogram, by sonar and/or by hysteroscopy. Its treatment involves abdominal surgery with the surgical removal of the tumor. The operation is called a *myomectomy*. (See Figure 6.1.)

If the parts forming the uterus, prior to birth, do not properly grow together, then the woman is born with a wall, either complete or incomplete within the uterine cavity. The presence of a septum within the uterine cavity may result in infertility but more often results in repeated miscarriages. Here again, the only treatment is surgical. The most common approach is that of performing abdominal surgery. Here the uterus is opened and the wall cut out. The uterus is then sutured closed and the abdominal surgery completed in the conventional manner. In about 70% of the cases a woman who has had such a procedure is able to conceive and carry on uneventfully. Since this surgery produces a scar in the uterine wall which may represent a potential weakened area, most obstetricians are reluctant to allow such a uterus to be subjected to the stresses of labor. For this reason most women who have had uterine surgery producing a uterine scar, whether performed for the removal of a fibroid or the excision of a septum, are delivered by Cesarean section. (See Figure 6.2.)

Fallopian tube reconstructive surgery involves a surgical attempt to restore the anatomy of a Fallopian tube. The Fallopian tube is a muscular, movable tubal structure which at one end is connected to the uterus and at the other end forms a funnel-like structure called the *fimbria*. The outer surface of the Fallopian tube is covered with a

Fallopian Tube

143

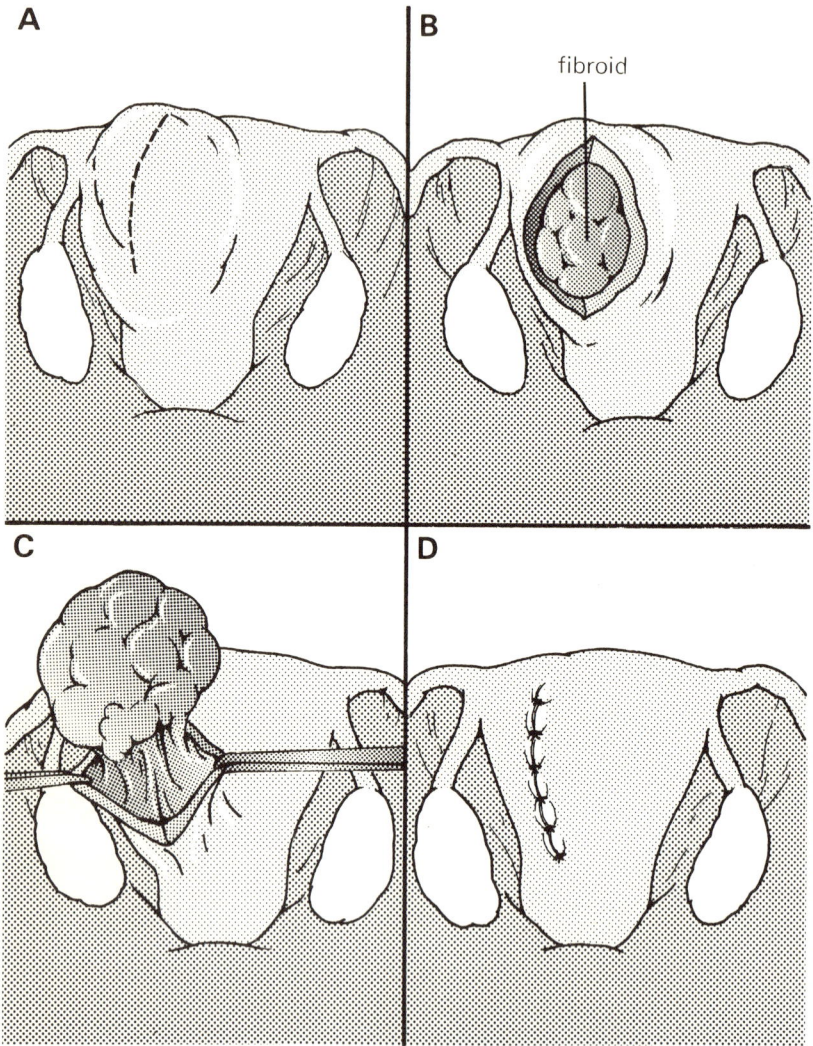

Figure 6.1 *Myomectomy. When it is appropriate, a fibroid may be surgically removed from the uterus and the defect closed.*

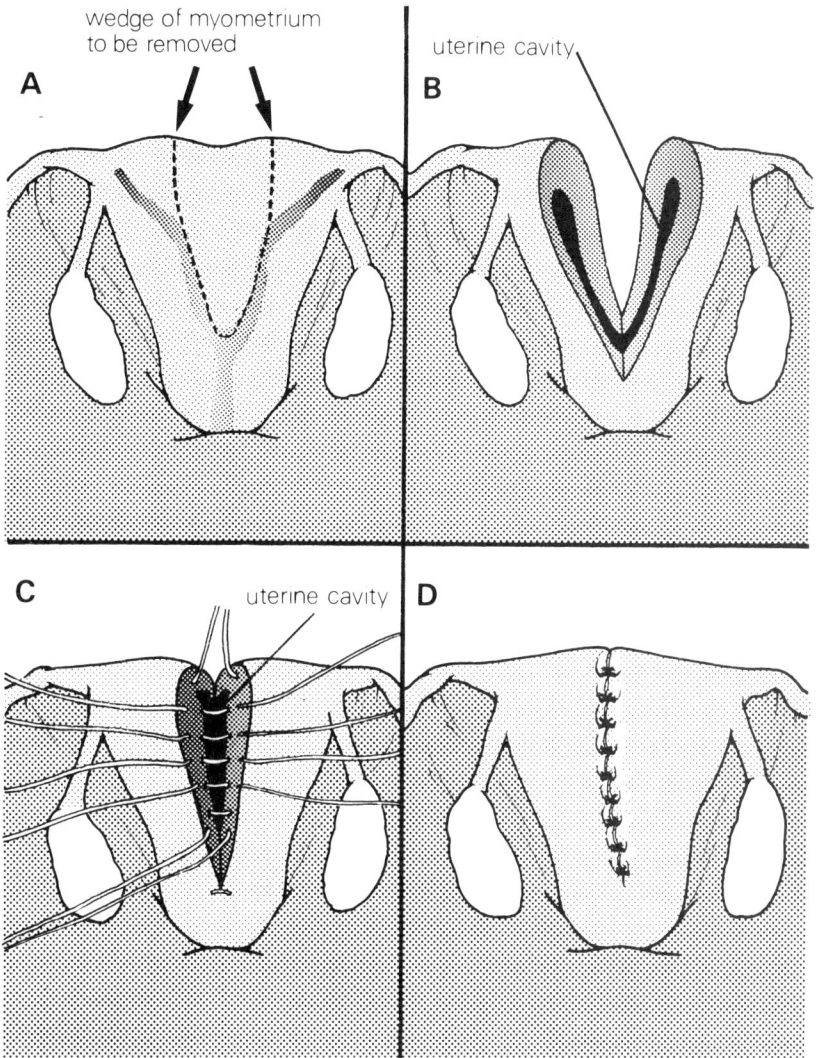

Figure 6.2 *The removal of a septum from a uterus*
  A. *The uterus containing the septum.*
  B. *Cutting out the septum.*
  C. *Sewing the uterus closed.*
  D. *The reconstructed uterus.*

slippery membrane called the *peritoneum*. The inner channel of the Fallopian tube is covered with a multifolded lining with many tiny moving hair-like projections called the *cilia*. This lining, the *endosalpinx*, produces a fluid secretion. The contraction of the muscular layer of the tube, the beating of the hair-like cilia and the movement of the fluid all combine to move the sperm and the egg through the Fallopian tube.

If scar tissue forms around the outside surface of the tube the movement of this tube and the ability of the fimbria to pick up an egg is drastically reduced. The surgical solution for this is to cut away the scar tissue allowing free movement of the tube. If all structures are normal after the surgical procedure, if the Fallopian tube is left totally undamaged, then the probability of becoming pregnant and achieving delivery is quite good, of the order of 70–80%.

Lysis of Adhesions

The procedure, called *lysis of adhesions*, may be done by using laparoscopy. Laparoscopy involves inserting a telescope-like device through the navel and visualizing the abdominal contents. If the tubes are found to be covered with very thin web-like adhesive bands, an additional instrument can be inserted to cut away and break up these bands. If the bands of connective tissue are more dense, using laparoscopy or culdoscopy becomes prohibitive and dangerous. Instead, a lower abdominal incision can be made and the abdomen entered as for regular surgery. Here, the scar tissue bands are cut away and the abdomen closed. (See Figures 6.3 and 6.4.)

An obstruction within the channel of the tube, blocking the tube, can only be corrected by surgically *excising* (cutting away) that segment of the

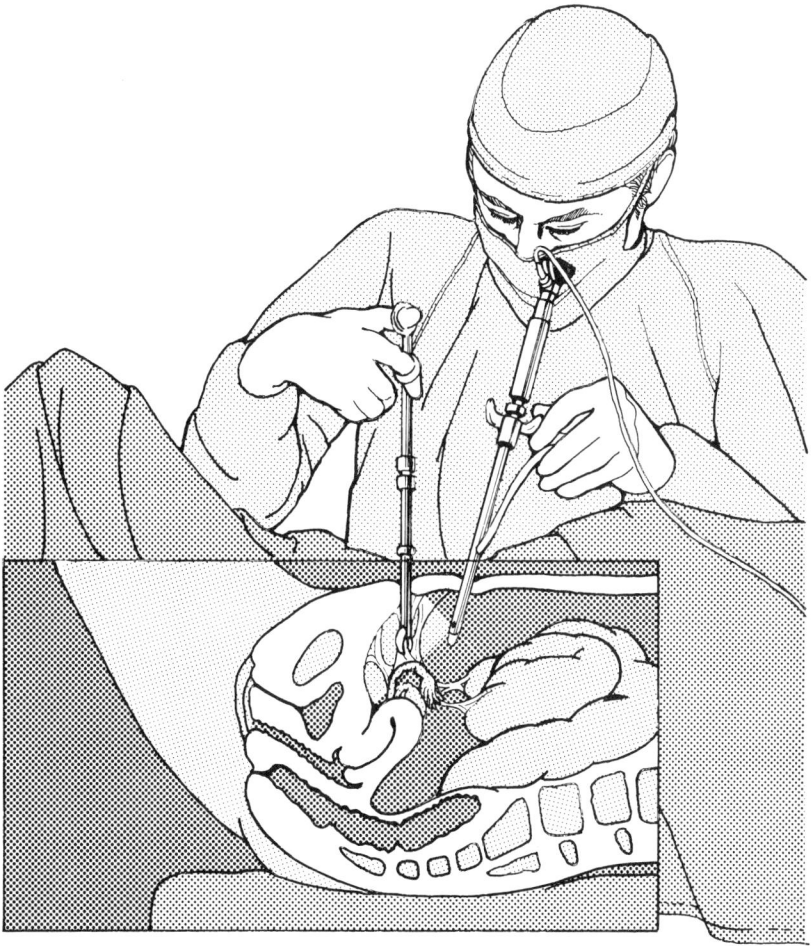

Figure 6.3 *Cutting adhesions with laparoscopic instrument and under laparoscopic observation.*

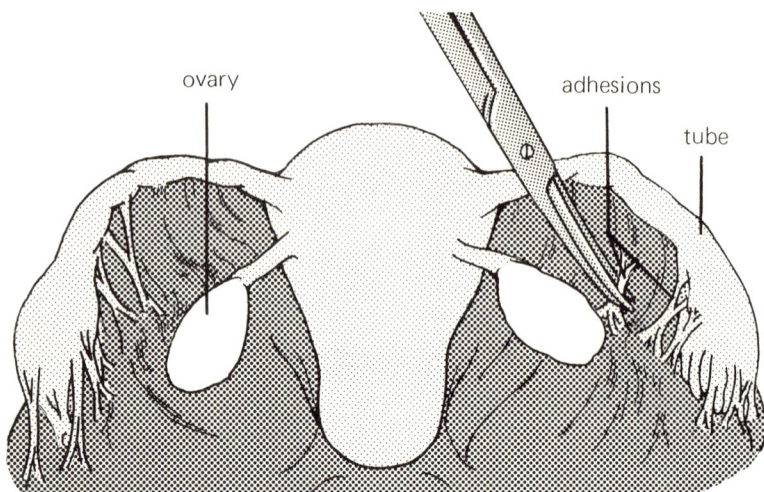

Figure 6.4 *Adhesions being cut away.*

tube that is blocked and then anastomosing (rejoining) the healthy tube segments. This procedure of removing a portion of tube and then rejoining the remaining portions is called *excision and anastomosis*. This is probably one of the most exciting areas of infertility surgery at this time. Recent advances in this area, using very fine suture and a microscope have significantly improved the results of such surgery. Though the technique of *microsurgery*, which entails using fine suture, careful tissue handling and manipulation under a microscope, is still a new technique it is very promising. The success rate in terms of live births using microsurgery compared to regular tubal surgery is approximately twice. The live birth rate, using microsurgery to reverse a previous tubal ligation, a female sterilization procedure, in selected cases is approximately 65%. The live birth rate

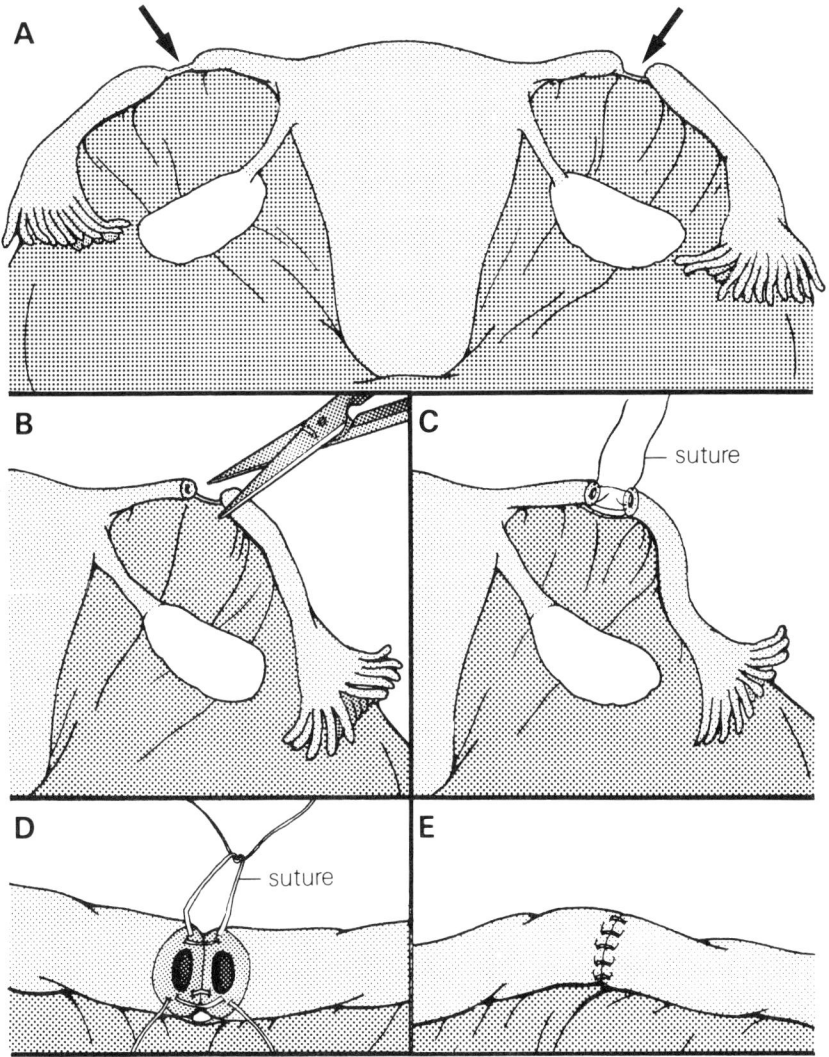

Figure 6.5 *Technique of reversal of a tubal ligation. The obstructed segment of each tube is cut out and the tube segments sewn back together (anastomosis).*

149

using conventional surgery to rejoin tubes previously ligated is approximately 30%. (See Figure 6.5.)

If an obstruction is at the mid-portion of the Fallopian tube, that area that is obstructed can be cut away and the tube rejoined using microsurgery. If the obstruction is at the junction of the Fallopian tube to the uterus, here too the obstruction can be cut away and microsurgical technique used to rejoin the tube to the surface of the uterus. If the obstruction is within the wall of the uterus at the point where the tube enters the uterus, then the Fallopian tube must be reimplanted into the uterine wall. Each of these procedures is associated with its own success rate, and the success rate depends upon the surgical techniques and the amount of damage done to the Fallopian tube.

Tubal
Reimplantation

The most significant lesion in the Fallopian tube is an obstruction to the fimbria. A chronic inflammatory process can cause the fimbria, the funnel-shaped structure at the end of the tube to become stuck together. The tube becomes enlarged, forming essentially a bag of fluid. The lining of the tube may become irreversibly damaged. The folds of this tissue may become destroyed and the hair-like cilia permanently removed. The muscles within the Fallopian tube may be destroyed and scar tissue will grow in its place. The result is that all the structures needed to allow an egg to be picked up and moved along the tube are destroyed. A severely scarred mid-portion of the tube may be removed and the tube rejoined but, if the end of the tube is scarred there is no way of substituting for it. As of today, in spite of a great deal of work there is no artificial device that can be used that can replace the fimbria or the entire Fallopian tube itself. The blunted sack-like end of the tube may be opened by one of a variety of surgical procedures and sutured in an open position. Occasionally, some regeneration (regrowth) of the lining tissue may occur, and pregnancy does follow. The pregnancy rate following such fimbrial surgery, known as *salpingostomy*, is approximately 15–30%. (See Figure 6.6.)

Salpingostomy

The consideration of Fallopian tube surgery must not be taken lightly. All surgery is associated with some risk. With Fallopian tube surgery, failure of the surgery does not simply mean that the woman will not become pregnant. Another complication may exist. The patient may indeed become pregnant, but instead of that pregnancy being within the uterus, the fertilized egg may be trapped within the Fallopian tube and the pregnancy will remain and grow within the tube. This is known as a *tubal pregnancy*. This is a potentially dangerous situation because as the pregnancy grows, the tube may be torn and sudden abdominal bleeding may occur. The amount and the degree of bleeding may be such that the patient may be thrown into sudden shock or even may die. When considering tubal surgery the risks and the benefits must be weighed carefully. The extreme desire to bear a child must be weighed against the risks of tubal pregnancy. It is nevertheless true that most pregnancies that occur following tubal surgery occur in the uterus and not in the Fallopian tube. As techniques improve, the incidence of tubal pregnancy decreases.

Endometriosis is a condition in which the tissue which is usually found lining the uterine cavity, is also found outside the uterus. Since this material is very irritating to its surrounding normal tissue it

Endometriosis

151

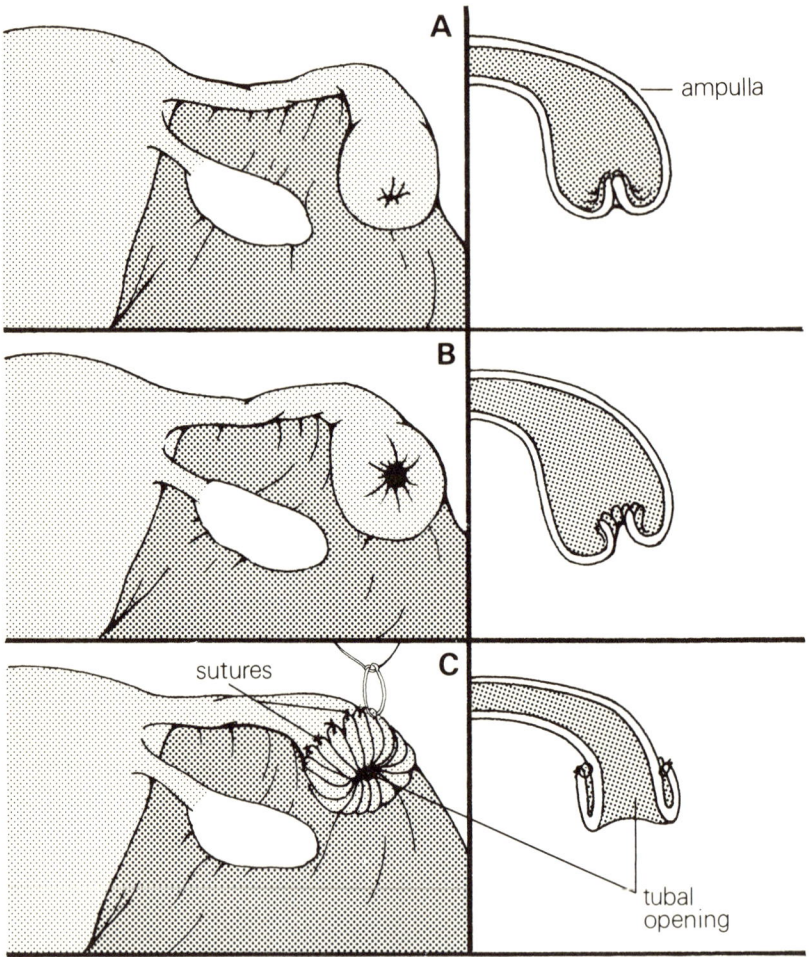

Figure 6.6 *Salpingostomy. A hydrosalpinx may be surgically opened and its anatomy reconstructed. This procedure is known as a* salpingostomy.

    A. *The hydrosalpinx before being opened.*

    B. *The clubbed end is carefully opened along the natural folds of the tissue.*

    C. *The fimbria are then everted, like the petals of a flower, and sewn into position.*

may cause pain, scarring and infertility. Endometriosis as a cause of infertility has been reviewed in Chapter 4. At this point its therapy will be discussed. Endometriosis may be treated medically, by giving drugs, and/or surgically, by actually cutting away or burning the areas of endometriosis.

Before any treatment is begun, the woman suspected of having endometriosis usually has endoscopy performed, be it culdoscopy or laparoscopy. This procedure allows the physician to directly observe the abdominal contents and examine them for endometriosis by means of a telescope inserted into the body. It permits the examining doctor to confirm his clinical impression and to see the extent and the amount of scarring the endometriosis has caused. From this, the proper mode of therapy can be selected. If there are large ovarian cysts called *endometriomas*, filled with endometriosis, or if there is extensive spread with much scarring, surgery may be the preferred treatment. On the other hand, if there is a small amount of endometriosis then medical therapy may be used.

The tissue comprising the areas of endometriosis depends upon the presence of estrogen for its growth. If the effect of estrogen could be diminished or if the actual amount of estrogen produced in the patient's body could be reduced temporarily then the areas of endometriosis would shrivel up. The object of medical therapy is to produce just such a state. This can be accomplished by using one of several drugs – Danocrine (Danazol), Provera (medroxyprogesterone), or oral contraceptives given in a non-cyclic manner. The chosen drug is given daily for about a six month period. The exact duration of treatment may vary depending on the extent of the disease and the response to therapy. The areas of endometriosis shrink to small areas of scar tissue many times smaller than their pre-treatment size. If the endometriosis was surrounded by scar tissue and adhesions, these scars will remain after medical therapy and may continue to prevent conception. They can only be treated surgically.

Surgical treatment involves entering the abdomen and removing each area of endometriosis. The defects created are carefully closed with fine suture material. Then the abdomen is closed.

The two modes of therapy may be combined. A woman may receive a course of medical therapy before surgery to shrink the affected areas and thus simplify the operation. On the other hand, a woman who has had surgery may be placed on medication to ensure the complete removal of every trace of endometriosis. Medical therapy alone in selected cases can offer successful treatment and pregnancy. Medical therapy and surgical therapy combined or alone can deal effectively with endometriosis.

Polycystic Ovary Syndrome

Polycystic ovary syndrome is a particular kind of anovulation in which the ovaries develop many small cysts and become enlarged. In an extreme form known as *Stein-Leventhal Syndrome*, the affected women become obese and develop a masculinized hair distribution. Polycystic ovary syndrome, referred to as "PCO Syndrome" by its friends and acquaintances, can be treated like any form of anovulation. In properly selected cases, after a complete infertility evaluation the woman

Medical Therapy

may be considered for Clomiphene therapy. If ovulation fails to occur, Clomiphene and HCG treatment may be given. If this is unsuccessful then Clomiphene, Pergonal (HMG) and HCG treatment may be used. Some physicians may consider the use of Pergonal (HMG) and HCG for those patients who did not ovulate on the therapy described thus far.

If all of these forms of treatment are unsuccessful or if the physician feels that the use of Pergonal is not appropriate for the patient then a surgical procedure called a *wedge resection* is considered. An ovarian wedge resection consists of removing a wedged-shaped segment from each ovary and then sewing closed the defect in the ovary. This procedure induces ovulation in women with PCO Syndrome by shifting the metabolism of the ovary. Medical treatment using Clomiphene is usually the first form of therapy chosen rather than a surgical approach. This is because about 80% of PCO patients treated medically will ovulate without the need for surgery. Furthermore, a significant percentage of women who have had wedge resections will develop adhesions around their ovaries and tubes. Though they may ovulate after surgery they may have difficulty becoming pregnant because of these adhesions. For these reasons a medical approach is usually chosen before a surgical one for Polycystic ovary syndrome. (See Figure 6.7.)

Surgical Therapy
i. Wedge Resection

Another means of therapy for infertile couples involves the use of artificial insemination. Artificial insemination is the introduction of sperm into the female reproductive tract using a syringe or other device, rather than using a penis. There are two forms of artificial insemination. A woman may have the sperm of her husband instilled within her vagina or may have the sperm of a different male inserted. In the first case the process is called *artificial*

III
ARTIFICIAL
INSEMINATION

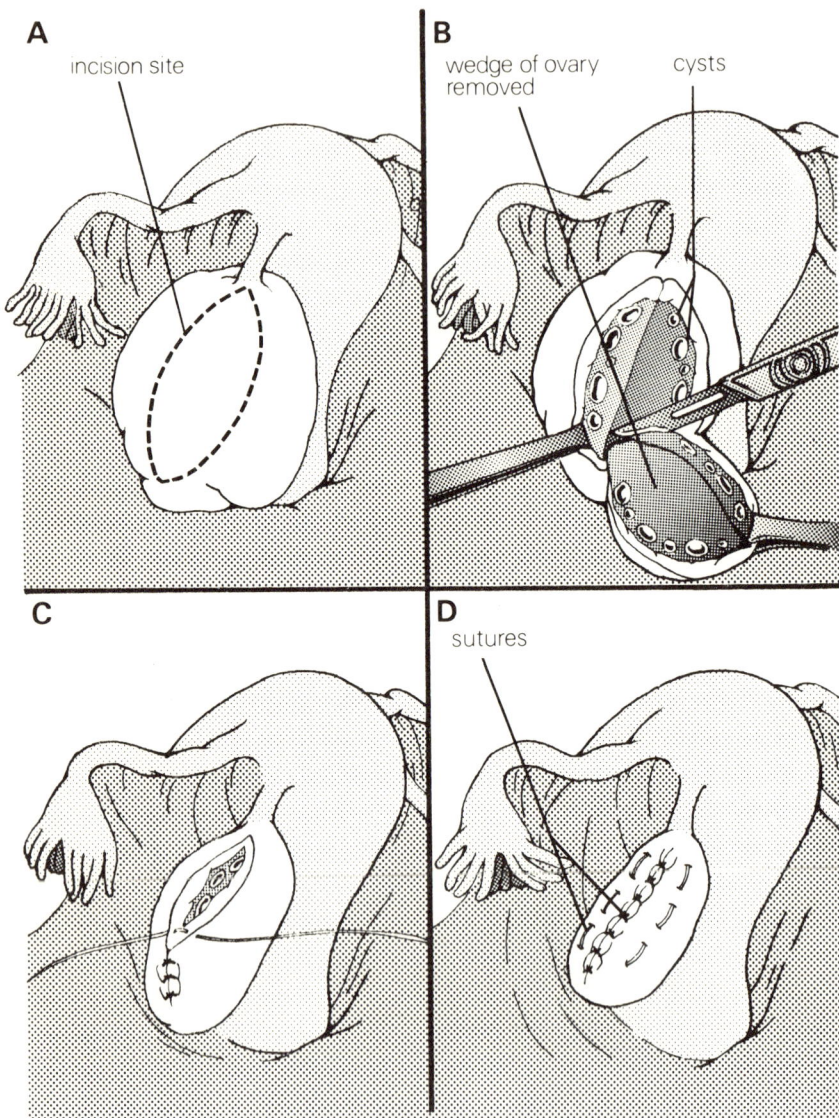

Figure 6.7 *Ovarian wedge resection. A wedge-shaped segment of ovary is removed and the ovary is then sewn closed.*

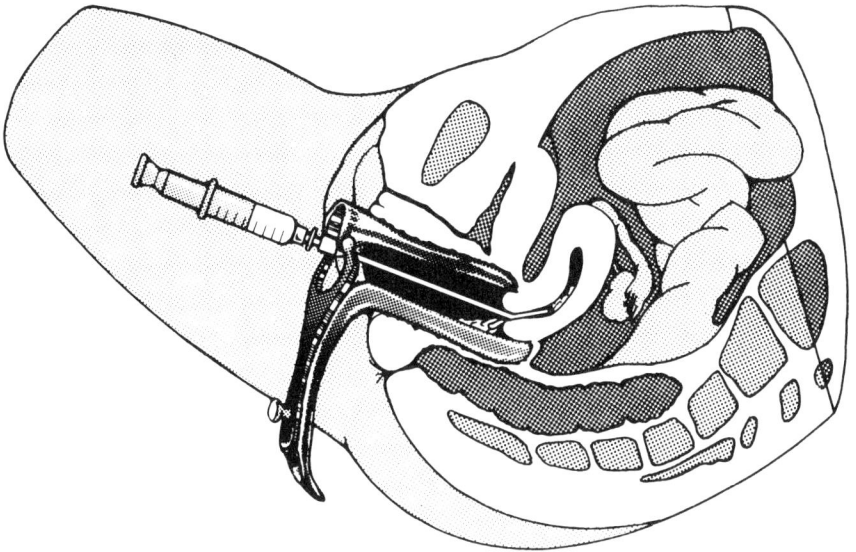

Figure 6.8 *Artificial insemination. Sperm is placed into the cervix or vagina using a syringe and a long tube.*

insemination – *homologous*, or *husband* and abbreviated as AIH. In the second case, the process is referred to as *artificial insemination - donor*, and is abbreviated to AID. AIH is used when a male is technically unable to instill his own sperm into the woman's vagina. This may be a result of an abnormality of the structure of his penis or an inability for the male sex partner to achieve sufficient rigidity of his penis to enter the vagina. It can also be used when there are cervical abnormalities such as antibody problems or stricture of the cervix. In this case the husband's sperm is not instilled within the vagina but is instilled directly into the uterine cavity. This procedure is known as *intrauterine* insemination. (See Figure 6.8.)

If the male is sterile and the female has no

AIH

AID

reproductive problems then donor artificial insemination can be used. In this case sperm obtained by masturbation from an unidentified male who has previously been screened to match the characteristics of the male sexual partner of the infertile couple is instilled within the vagina. Approximately 50% of couples using donor insemination achieve pregnancy. The success rate with AIH varies tremendously and depends upon the indication for the process.

IV
JOGGING AND
INFERTILITY

Of the various crazes to spread through the United States, the desire to improve one's physical fitness is probably the most reasonable and most welcome in years. The most recent development in this area is the extensive use of jogging, running and long-distance marathon running by both men and women. Its benefits to the cardio-vascular system appear to be beyond dispute though its projected effects on longevity still remain to be proven. Some discussion has revolved around the effect of running on the reproductive ability. Like many simply phrased questions the answer is complex. For most people running causes a loss in fatty tissue, among other things. In the human female, fatty tissue acts very much like an endocrine gland, converting some of the substances from the adrenal gland to estrogens. An obese woman has a large quantity of fatty tissue and therefore is producing a lot of extra estrogen. In a certain sense, this estrogen acts very much like a built-in birth control pill. It is perhaps for this reason that a significant percentage of very overweight women tend not to ovulate. If running results in weight loss and the reduction of total fat, then for these patients, running may be a very definite benefit. On the other hand, if it reduces the normal percentage of fat in the female body below a certain point, ovulation seems to become less likely. An important factor in long-distance running is the creation of a stress situation, causing the cardiac rate to increase and the heart muscle to exercise vigorously over an extended period of time. If running produces an overall stress situation the result may be a chronic stress anovulation. This stress anovulation is not a result of the increased load on the heart, but may be a manifestation of physiological stress or psychological stress in the central nervous system. Rapid fluctuations in weight may also produce an anovulatory state and this may very well follow jogging.

The point that is being made is that jogging may be very helpful to some women and may be detrimental to others. Though joggers are being studied in several institutions, there does not yet seem to be enough data to determine the percentage of women who stop ovulating after starting a jogging program and the percentage who were anovulatory who begin making eggs after starting jogging. It does seem clear however, that there is a small percentage of women who cease ovulating when a vigorous program of running has been instituted. The mechanism as outlined above, may be that of simple stress, weight fluctuation with loss or change in ratio of total body fat relative to total body mass. Whatever the mechanism involved, it does not seem to be a permanent change. Furthermore, there is no reason to believe at this time that women who are anovulatory following jogging will be any more difficult to treat than any anovulatory women. Clomiphene, or Clomiphene and HCG seem to be quite successful treatments. However, since no treatment is always better than even the most benign treatment I frequently suggest to those women who are joggers and who have become anovulatory after the beginning of their running, to stop jogging temporarily.

With the extensive use of oral contraceptives, it is not uncommon to hear of a woman who apparently does not ovulate and menstruate after stopping the use of "the pill." In medical terminology this is called *postpill amenorrhea.* Though it is spoken of frequently, postpill amenorrhea occurs in less than 1% of women who have used oral contraceptives. It is not related to the duration of the contraceptive use. Women who have used birth control pills for several months have the same incidence of postpill amenorrhea as those who have used the medication for years. Furthermore, as you will soon see, most cases of postpill amenorrhea may have little to do with oral contraceptive use.

Women who have postpill amenorrhea fall into three groups. The first is comprised of those who ovulated infrequently before starting oral contraceptives and continue to be anovulatory after stopping them. In this case the anovulation is the continuation of a previous menstrual pattern rather than being caused by birth control pills.

The second group is composed of women who had regular menses prior to birth control pill use but do not ovulate after stopping "the pill." However, it appears as if most of these women would have stopped ovulating even if they had not used oral contraceptives. This is demonstrated statistically by noting that the incidence of anovulation and infertility among non-pill users is the same as among those who used oral contraceptives. If birth control pills caused lasting anovulation there would be more amenorrhea and infertility in the group of ex-pill users. This is *not* the case.

The last group are those women whose ovulatory centers, in fact, may have remained suppressed after the use of oral contraceptives. The result is the failure to resume normal ovulation after birth control pills have been stopped. This group represents a very small percentage of all postpill amenorrhea patients.

It is very difficult to separate the second from the third group just mentioned. In a sense it is of little significance since members of all three groups can usually be treated equally well and successfully. The therapy for anovulation as discussed earlier in this chapter is used. Most women with postpill amenorrhea respond well to Clomiphene treatment.

And so we see that various forms of problems each have their own approach and their own degree of success. Anovulation can be treated with medication, inducing ovulation in approximately greater than 95% of cases and pregnancy in about 50% of those cases. Uterine reconstruction can be associated with approximately 70% live birth rate. Fallopian tube reconstruction is associated with approximately 15–65% live birth rate depending upon the location and degree of damage to the tube.

Not being able to become pregnant is not the only reproductive problem that requires attention. The next chapter will discuss miscarriage.

Chapter 7

Conception Is Not the Only Problem:
miscarriage

INFERTILITY IS THE inability of a couple to produce a pregnancy. But what do we say about couples who conceive, only to lose the conception early in pregnancy. Strictly speaking these people are not "infertile" because they can conceive. Nonetheless, if the losses are repetitive and not isolated events the result is the same as infertility – they are unable to have children.

Because "miscarriage" is a separate category from "infertility" it is presented here as a separate chapter. In most cases the diagnostic procedures and the treatments are the same or similar to those already presented in the diagnosis and treatment of infertility. Nevertheless, where appropriate these techniques will be briefly reviewed here to emphasize their use in the evaluation and therapy of miscarriage.

It is an extemely difficult and upsetting experience for two people who have just celebrated the joy of conception, to find that their pregnancy has not survived. Their questions are usually, "Why us?" "Why did it happen?" and "Will this happen again?" Let us begin by answering these questions.

It is difficult to tell any individual couple why

they lost their pregnancy. However, a certain number of general statements can be made that are still relevant.

The loss of a conception early in pregnancy is not at all an unusual phenomenon. Approximately 15–20% of all pregnancies are lost before the twenty-sixth week of pregnancy. In layman's language, such a loss of a conception is known as a *miscarriage*. In medical terminology, the loss of a fetus before the twenty-sixth week of pregnancy is termed an *abortion*. Note that the technical use of "abortion" does not imply that the loss of the fetus has resulted from manipulation or a surgical procedure as it does in layman's language. An abortion may be *induced*, meaning that it has resulted from some manipulation, or may be *spontaneous*, implying that nothing has been done to produce the loss of the pregnancy. Spontaneous abortion, i.e., a miscarriage, is the subject of the discussion in this chapter.

If a woman becomes pregnant and has a miscarriage it is very probable that this will be an isolated event. By this I mean that she will probably be able to conceive again, have an uneventful pregnancy and deliver a perfectly normal child. Most miscarriages are one time occurrences and, though an upsetting experience, should only temporarily interrupt a couple's reproductive plans. If a woman goes on to have a total of three consecutive miscarriages it is most likely that a definite problem exists and should be investigated. The latter condition, known as *habitual abortion*, deprives a couple of the ability to have their own children.

The first twelve weeks of pregnancy, known as the *first trimester*, is the time of greatest risk for mis-

II
INCIDENCE OF
MISCARRIAGE

III
DEFINITION
Miscarriage

Abortion

Induced
Spontaneous

Habitual

163

carriage, since 86% occur during this period.

If a conception is spontaneously and completely expelled from the uterus into the vagina leaving no residual pregnancy tissue in the uterine cavity, it is

Complete

known as a *complete abortion*. If some tissue is passed and the remainder is retained in the uterus,

Incomplete
Missed

this is referred to as an *incomplete abortion*. A *missed abortion* occurs when the pregnancy dies and all the tissue remains within the uterus. No treatment is usually required immediately after a verified complete abortion. On the other hand, a woman with an incomplete or missed abortion should have the tissue removed from the uterus. This is usually done by a minor surgical procedure known as a *dilation and curettage* or a *D & C*. In this procedure, the cervix, the opening of the uterus, is stretched and the lining of the cavity is scraped off or curetted. A D & C helps to diminish the chances of heavy vaginal bleeding and subsequent uterine infection.

IV
CAUSES

Most miscarriages are random mistakes of nature that usually do not repeat themselves. It is only when a woman has had three consecutive, spontaneous abortions that one should consider a

Single Miscarriage

complete medical evaluation. Before this time, after one or even two consecutive miscarriages, the most

Blighted Egg or
Blighted Preg-
nancy

likely explanation is that of a *blighted egg* or *blighted pregnancy*. In these instances, from the initial division of the fertilized egg, there is something grossly abnormal about the cells produced. This may be a result of a defective egg or sperm cell. In a kind of protective mechanism built into most animals, these grossly abnormal masses of cells rarely survive. It is a way of preventing the birth of markedly abnormal offspring. Many of these blighted pregnancies are lost so early that the patient may not even realize that she was pregnant. It is only by careful examination of the menstrual tissue that abnormal products of conception may be found. This condition is probably more common than is believed but is usually not a cause of repetitive miscarriage. A blighted pregnancy is a result of a chance abnormality in the development of an egg or a sperm which results in the abnormal pregnancy. It must be emphasized that in this case, both members of the couple are capable of producing normal cells in the vast majority of cases and that these mistakes of nature can occur in anyone without affecting further reproduction.

Habitual Abortion

If a woman loses three or more consecutive pregnancies she is said to have *habitual abortions.* This couple can achieve conception and therefore is not strictly "infertile." However, their efforts are unable to produce a living child. The problem may be related to genetic abnormality, hormonal problems, a uterine abnormality, cervical abnormality or T-mycoplasma infection.

Genetic Abnormality

Some men and women may carry an abnormal genetic information in their chromosomes. This defective hereditary material may not express itself in that particular individual but when it is combined with the genetic material from the partner of the couple, the result is a conception that cannot live. Certain genetic combinations and abnormalities are not consistent with the survival of a pregnancy. When a couple repetitively produces pregnancies which end in miscarriages, particularly within the first twelve weeks of pregnancy, one must seriously consider a *genetic abnormality.* In this case, as opposed to the blighted pregnancy situation described above, the couple is producing defective genetic material much of the time and not on rare occasions. Genetic studies, called *karyotyping*, must be done to diagnose such genetic problems and to tell the couple what the probability of their ever being able to produce a pregnancy that will survive.

Another cause of habitual abortion is the

Hormonal Abnormality

derangement in one of the hormonal systems of the woman's body. Since the female provides the intrauterine environment for the pregnancy, any significant biochemical disturbance of this environment may seriously affect the viability of the fetus.

Thyroid

Overfunctioning or underfunctioning of the thyroid gland can lead to a loss of pregnancy. Similarly,

Adrenal Gland
Diabetes

abnormal functioning of the adrenal gland can also result in a miscarriage. If the woman is a diabetic who is not under control, the conception may be lost early or at any time right through to the end of pregnancy. Diabetics must be managed very carefully

Progesterone

during their pregnancies. A progesterone deficiency that is not significant enough to prevent pregnancy may exist and be just severe enough to allow the loss of a new conception. The diagnoses of any of these hormonal abnormalities can be made by taking a blood sample and testing it for the appropriate hormonal products. In screening for diabetes, a glucose tolerance test would be most appropriate.

Uterine Structural Abnormality

In the process of development the fertilized egg implants on the lining of the uterine cavity and then progressively enlarges in size. The conception depends upon the blood supply in the uterine wall below the area of implantation for its nourishment. It also depends upon the uterine cavity to offer a protected space into which it can grow. If the blood supply to the developing conception is diminished or if the pregnancy must compete for growing space in the uterus then a miscarriage may result. Abnormalities in the structure of the uterine wall may do exactly this.

The uterus may contain a non-cancerous tumor known as a *myoma* or a *fibroid*. Such a tumor may *Fibroid* be entirely within the uterine wall or may project into the uterine cavity. If the fertilized egg implants on the tumor the tissue is not capable of supplying a sufficient blood supply to sustain the growing pregnancy. Furthermore, as the conception grows, so will the fibroid. Often the tumor will compress the uterine cavity providing insufficient room for the growing pregnancy. Thus, by impairing the blood supply and/or reducing the uterine cavity space, the fibroid is capable of producing a miscarriage. However, the presence of such a tumor does not necessarily mean that it is the cause of the abortions. It is possible for the fibroid to be on the outside surface of the uterus without affecting the pregnancy. The uterus must be studied by one of the techniques to be mentioned below to determine if the fibroid is related to the miscarriages.

Occasionally a woman will have a uterus that *Septum* appears perfectly normal on the outside but has a wall projecting into the cavity on the inside. Such a wall is known as a *uterine septum* and can act just as the fibroid to produce miscarriages.

The diagnosis of any abnormality of the uterine cavity is usually begun by performing an x-ray called a *hysterosalpingogram*. The uterus, which is made of soft tissue, will not show up on x-ray. However, if the cavity is filled with a fluid that can be seen on x-ray, then one is capable of photographing a silhouette of the uterine cavity. Any change of the usual triangular shape of the space may be a result of compression by a fibroid or a uterine septum.

The surface of the uterine cavity can be directly visualized by placing a telescope-like device, called a *hysteroscope*, through the vagina and cervix into the uterus. This way the fibroid or septum can actually be seen rather than relying on a photograph of a silhouette as with an x-ray. Both of these techniques have been discussed in greater detail in Chapter 5.

Incompetent Cervical Os

As the fetus grows it exerts greater pressure on the opening of the uterus, the cervix. Circular muscle and connective tissue fibers present within the body of the cervix keep it closed and the pregnancy within the uterine cavity. If these tissue fibers are defective, then the cervix is unable to maintain its closed state against the downward pressure of the uterine contents. When this happens, the cervix opens and the pregnancy is passed out into the vagina and the outer world well before it is capable of surviving on its own. This condition is known as an *incompetent cervical os*. The history of a previous miscarriage can make the physician suspicious that a woman has an incompetent os. The patient with this problem classically describes the painless loss of the pregnancy as opposed to experiencing the cramps of labor usually felt with other forms of miscarriages. It can be verified by performing a dilatation and curettage and actually feeling the kind of resistance the cervical tissue offers to manipulation.

T-mycoplasma

T-mycoplasma, an organism between a virus and a bacteria, has been cited by some as being a cause of habitual abortion. This is still controversial and is mentioned at this time for the sake of completeness. It remains for the future for more definitive work to be uncovered.

Note that in the discussion of the causes of miscarriage, physical or emotional trauma has not been mentioned. It is not uncommon for a woman to lose a pregnancy and then feel that it is a result of something that she did. She may feel that she engaged in too much activity, that she worried too much or that she had too much or too little exercise. She may wonder if that extra long automobile trip had anything to do with her miscarriage. Indeed, most of these things are truly irrelevant. The intrauterine environment is a very safe, self-contained fluid medium that is able to sustain tremendous shock. A normally functioning placenta is able to biochemically maintain the needs of a normal fetus. If the environmental stress of every day activity is enough to upset the balance of the fetus, then one must consider the basic situation so compromised that survival was almost impossible from the beginning. There is no need for individuals or couples to torture themselves with feelings of guilt because of a loss of pregnancy. In most cases there was nothing that they did that produced the miscarriage.

Now that the causes of miscarriage have just been reviewed, let us turn to its treatment. Since a single miscarriage is usually not associated with any further reproductive problems a full evaluation is usually not carried out. For the same reason no treatment is given.

The woman who has had habitual abortions and a hormonal problem diagnosed should have blood tests performed to determine thyroid and

**V
NON-CAUSES**

**VI
TREATMENT
Single
Miscarriage**

**Habitual
Abortion**

169

Hormonal Problem

progesterone levels and adrenal gland function. If these studies reveal a hormonal problem then the woman should be given those particular deficient substances. If she has a thyroid deficiency, thyroid medication should be considered. There are several drugs that may be given. The physician will select the most appropriate medication. If the adrenal glands are not working up to normal levels, one of the corticosteroid drugs will be selected and given. For progesterone deficiency, the use of Clomiphene or progesterone has already been discussed. Please note that Clomiphene is not given during pregnancy, but may be considered before it.

Uterine Structural Problem

If a hysterosalpingogram and/or hysteroscopy reveals an abnormality of the uterine contour such as a fibroid or a uterine septum, these abnormalities should be removed. An abdominal surgical procedure is necessary to accomplish this. There are several techniques that can be used for the removal of the uterine septum. The procedure is basically that of opening the uterus, cutting out the septum or fibroid and then sewing the uterine wall back together again. For the removal of a fibroid, an incision is made into the wall of the uterus and the fibroid is extracted. The uterine wall defect is then closed. This procedure is known as a *myomectomy*.

Incompetent Cervix

The patient that is found to have an incompetent cervix as diagnosed by history and confirmed by performing a dilatation and curettage may have a *Shirodkar procedure* performed. In this procedure a heavy suture material is placed around the cervix, under the covering mucosal tissue. The suture is tied and acts as a substitute for the defective or missing connective tissue. The suture material actually ties the cervix in a closed, normal position. The

Shirodkar procedure may be done either before pregnancy or just after the patient has become pregnant, around the beginning of the second trimester.

If a reason for miscarriage is considered to be a T-mycoplasma infection, the couple should be treated with an appropriate antibiotic such as Doxycycline.

T-mycoplasma

Even though a single cause for habitual abortion may be found the remainder of the studies should still be completed. There is a certain small chance that a given couple may have multiple causes for their miscarriages. If treatment is to be successful all of the problems must be defined and corrected.

The causes and treatments for miscarriages have just been discussed. A single miscarriage, a spontaneous abortion, is usually an isolated non-recurring event, due to a blighted pregnancy. Since the couple is usually able to continue their reproductive lives having children as if nothing had occurred, no treatment is necessary. The couple that has three or more consecutive miscarriages is said to have habitual abortions. This is usually associated with one of several causes of miscarriage and unless treated the couple may very well be unable to establish a family. The methods of diagnosis and the appropriate therapy have been discussed.

Habitual abortion, like other problems in Reproductive Medicine, is being studied in many centers throughout the world. Many advances are expected in the near future both in diagnosis and treatment. The next chapter will discuss what can be expected from the Infertility research currently underway.

Chapter 8

The Future:
new solutions around the corner

INFERTILITY RESEARCH is progressing very rapidly. In the last fifteen to twenty years we have seen patients who were anovulators, (women who were unable to ovulate), successfully treated. Today, over 95% of the patients who are treated for anovulation will ovulate. This is just the most recent and tangible result of aggressive infertility research. The whole field is ripening, like a follicle ready to release its egg, ready to explode and generate new life in the very near future. In this chapter I will allow myself a bit of license and attempt to sketch for you the near future of Reproductive Medicine to show you what today's laboratory work will probably give us.

**I
TUBAL
PREGNANCY
SURGERY**

When a fertilized egg gets trapped in the tube instead of traveling into the uterus the result is known as a *tubal pregnancy*. The fertilized egg grows and stretches the tube until the wall begins to tear and then finally ruptures. The torn tube wall can bleed quite heavily and the woman may collapse or even die because of sudden blood loss.

The accepted treatment of tubal pregnancy is to operate and remove the tube containing the pregnancy. Unfortunately, no way has been found to

172

save the developing embryo and transplant it to allow its survival. It has been found that the removal of one tube can significantly reduce the chances of a woman becoming pregnant again. Because of this, an operation has been developed at our institution that can be used in selected cases to preserve the affected tube rather than removing it. The result appears to be the preservation of fertility.

The procedure involves the surgical removal of the affected portion of the Fallopian tube with an anastomosis (a reconnecting) of the remaining segments. In other words, the physician, who is an experienced microsurgeon, removes the portion of the oviduct containing the pregnancy and sews the two severed ends of the tube back together. The procedure uses very fine suture material to sew the tube and is done under a microscope. The technique has been used on only a few patients thus far including three women who had only one tube – the one containing the tubal pregnancy. The conventional treatment for these women would have been the removal of the tube containing the pregnancy and that would have made them sterile. Each patient who has had this procedure and who has desired to conceive has become pregnant, including the three women who each had one tube. This new approach to the treatment of tubal pregnancy is very promising and is the basis of continued work. It is hoped that in the future all tubal pregnancies can be saved and that no tube will have to be removed.

The function of the Fallopian tube is to offer an environment in which an egg may be fertilized and to carry the egg into the uterus. If the structure of the tube is somehow damaged it can no longer function properly. One of the most difficult problems for

**II
TRANSPLANTS**

the infertility specialist to deal with today is that of the severely scarred or deformed Fallopian tube. If the damage is bad enough no form of reconstructive surgery currently available can be effective at restoring the ability to conceive. The possibility of replacing poorly functioning tissue with artificial structures such as plastic tubes has been considered but so far has not been very helpful. And so, a woman with totally scarred Fallopian tubes or absent tubes cannot look forward to their substitution by an artificial tube. However, one area of very promising research is that of organ transplantation. The possibility of giving a woman a new Fallopian tube, a new ovary, or a male a new testis, is something that must be thought of very seriously.

Fallopian Tubes

A source of Fallopian tubes for women already exists in that population of patients who desire surgical sterilization. Fallopian tube transplants have been done successfully in rabbits, pigs and sheep. And though human Fallopian tube transplantations have been attempted in women, they have been unsuccessful in the sense that pregnancies have not occurred in any of these patients. But it appears certain that in the very near future the technical problems will be eliminated and those women with irreparably damaged Fallopian tubes will have somewhere to turn.

Uterus

Similarly, a woman without a uterus because of a congenital abnormality or a surgical procedure will be able to receive the uterus of a woman who has completed her childbearing and would now like to assist others in reproduction. Those women who have had premature ovarian failure or have been born with ovaries that fail to produce eggs for a variety of reasons, may be able to consider receiving

Ovary

an ovary from another woman. The possibility of receiving an ovarian transplant is something that is currently being investigated. It has been demonstrated to work in dogs but its success and safety in humans is yet to be proven. Nevertheless, there seems to be no question that as transplantation techniques improve and surgical approaches evolve, ovarian transplantation will become a reality.

Some have questioned whether or not a child born of a woman who has had an ovarian transplant can indeed be considered her child rather than the child of the donor. Though asking such questions at this time is premature, they will have to be asked eventually. I bring up this problem to stir your imagination and to point out that not all the problems of infertility are scientific. My own personal opinion is that the intrauterine environment and the care and nurturing of the newborn contribute at least as much to the development of the child as does the genetic material from the donated ovary. Therefore, I feel the mother has every right to consider the child born following an ovarian transplant to be hers rather than the child of the tissue donor.

The transplantation of tissue will certainly not be reserved for the human female. The human male is an excellent candidate for testicular transplantation. Indeed, a testicular transplant performed between identical twins has already been successfully completed. Thus, we know that the surgical expertise for this procedure already exists. The only problem that must still be solved is the technique of transplanting tissue between two non-related patients. Just as questions arise in the case of who is the parent

Testes

following ovarian transplant, the tissue donor or recipient, the same questions arise following testicular transplantation. One may ask whether or not the father of the child produced following testicular transplantation is the donor of the testis or the recipient of the testis. This problem becomes a bit more involved but precedence for this, in the case of artificial insemination, already exists.

**III
IN VITRO
FERTILIZA-
TION AND
EMBRYO
TRANSFER**

Tubal transplantation is not the only way of allowing a woman with irreparably scarred oviducts to become pregnant. An egg, ready to be released by the ovary, can be removed from the female body and fertilized outside the body in a laboratory. The fertilized egg is then allowed to divide and grow for about two days and then is implanted within the uterus of the same woman. Continued development is just as it would be during an ordinary pregnancy. This procedure is called *in vitro fertilization* and *embryo transfer*. This means that instead of waiting for an egg to be picked up and fertilized in a non-functioning Fallopian tube, the process is allowed to take place outside the body. The need for the tube is completely by-passed. This procedure has been done successfully in animals for years. It is currently being done experimentally in humans in the United Kingdom. The first verified human pregnancy and term delivery following this procedure has recently been announced. However, at this time there is no clinical information as to what these babies and adults will be like. There is insufficient information to date to allow this technique to be used in routine clinical practice. Nevertheless, I am sure that in the near future, *in vitro* fertilization with embryo transfer will be a therapeutic technique used in clinical practice for the treatment of infertility.

In vitro fertilization and embryo transfer can also provide a means of offering a pregnancy to a woman who is not only missing Fallopian tubes but may also be missing a uterus. For this woman, it is possible to remove an egg from her ovary, fertilize it with her husband's sperm in a laboratory apparatus and insert the fertilized ovum inside the uterus of another woman. In this case the fertilized egg will develop into an embryo and then a fetus in the uterus of someone else. When the time for delivery occurs, this woman, the *surrogate mother*, will **Surrogate Mother** deliver the child and the child will be raised by the woman whose egg was used. Not only can one soon foresee a new mode of therapy for a woman without a uterus and tubes, but one can imagine the development of a new occupation – the surrogate mother. Though this may seem bizarre to some and highly distasteful and disturbing to others, one must remember that this can offer a child to a highly motivated couple where no other alternatives are currently open. Furthermore, this child, unlike one resulting from adoption, will truly be a product of the reproductive material of both members of the couple.

Some who have heard and read of *in vitro* fertilization and embryo transplantation say that it is reminiscent of the hatcheries described in *Brave New World*. They fear that we are entering a time where humans will be manufactured in vast factories, controlled and manipulated for socio-political needs. They see the use of *in vitro* fertilization as the beginning of the ultimate corruption of mankind and so some have called for the termination of *in vitro* fertilization research. Is this the beginning of a *Brave New World* or the ultimate treatment for couples with currently insurmountable infertility problems?

The question can only be answered by the future. Like all things from stones to atomic energy, *in vitro* fertilization is neither good nor bad by itself. It is only its use that determines whether it is good or bad. In my opinion it would be wrong to stop the current work in *in vitro* fertilization. The result would be to stop progress and to deprive couples of children for fear that someone will pervert the use of this medical technique.

**IV
CLONING**

Recently, there has been much discussion of *cloning* and its significance to humans. It remains to be seen whether or not a successful human clone has been produced. However, it appears certain that if it has not already been done, it will be done in the future.

In my opinion, cloning does not truly offer a solution for the infertile couple. A clone is an exact, genetic duplicate of a single individual. A child is a product of the genetic material of two different individuals, truly the product of a union of two people. The usual desire of a couple wishing to conceive a pregnancy is to produce a wonderful new individual who is original, and who reflects aspects of each of its parents, and not that of making a carbon copy of one of the members of the couple. It is not clear then that cloning will offer a satisfactory answer to the couple. Its role in the socio-political development of our societies remains to be defined. The possibilities of both good and bad are staggering.

The investigational work described thus far has been of a surgical nature. It would be wrong to give you the impression that this is the only kind of research being done. Some very interesting work in the development of new drugs is being carried on at this time.

A substance known as *Gonadotropin Releasing Hormone* or GnRH was discovered in the hypothalamus and was found to control the release of the hormones LH and FSH by the pituitary. By giving GnRH to certain anovulatory women the release of an egg from the ovary would result. Unfortunately, GnRH must be given by frequent injection to be effective, thus it is not a practical drug.

Laboratory work is currently underway to change the structure of synthetic GnRH so that it can be given more easily and less frequently. This is called constructing *hormone analogues*. It is hoped that a drug that can be given once daily, by mouth instead of by frequent injection will be made. The result would be a very effective, easily administerable medication. Recent findings make it appear that success is close at hand.

This has been a brief look into the near future. The possibilities are exciting and many. The results of current research will be conception for those couples who are considered untreatable today. At this moment there is no question in my mind that the advances I have just outlined will come to pass. The question is, "how soon?" The only thing more exciting than imagining what the future will bring, is working in an area of medical research that will actually produce these advances.

**V
HORMONE
ANALOGUES**

179

Chapter 9

Closing Thoughts

THE TITLE OF THIS chapter is "closing thoughts," rather than "final thoughts." I want to present some extraneous ideas at this point in the book because they do not fit easily into any of the categories discussed thus far. They are not the final thoughts on the subject of infertility. In fact, if there is one thing that I want to emphasize very strongly it is that there are no final thoughts about infertility. Reproductive medicine is making gains at an incredible rate. In writing the text of this book I have revised it several times just on the basis of progress made during the last several months. There is no question in my mind that in the very near future, patients who are considered very difficult to treat will be therapeutic successes. The future can only hold good news and more hope of a child for almost every couple who desires one. Do not give up your efforts in any way.

While going through the diagnostic procedures to discover the reason for your infertility, it is very important that you share your feelings with your physician and with each other. The inability to produce a child when you desire it strains the very fibers of the relationship of two people.

In past times of stress each of you has been able to turn to your partner to seek and gain emotional support. When fertility problems arise, a man and woman may begin to question each other's role in their predicament. Instead of being members of a couple they may become adversaries. There is a tendency for individual members of an infertile couple not to discuss their emotions. The result is an increasing feeling of isolation, frustration, hostility and depression. To help overcome this, make your physician a partner to your mind. Both of you confide in him and share your problems with him. Convert a tendency toward isolation into constant dialogue and sharing of feelings.

Infertility is a symptom of a medical problem. If you had a different medical problem such as a broken arm or an ulcer, you would not be reluctant to express your feelings about it. Similarly, ideally, there should be no difference in the feelings felt by an infertile couple. However, because the problem involves one's own sexuality, one's self-value, one's ego, the response is quite different. It takes a conscious effort for a man and a woman to share their feelings on this emotionally charged subject with each other and with a third person. Yet, if this effort is made, the benefits are enormous. Pressure and stress become diffused and though the problem itself may not be cured immediately, tolerating it, becomes much easier.

Fifteen percent of couples of reproductive age living in the United States are unable to bear children. This means that in any group of twenty couples there is bound to be at least one who is infertile. Though you may feel isolated at times, you are certainly not alone. In reaching out, you will find that there are many, many people who are willing and able to help you. Besides medical assistance, there are also groups offering counseling and general support. Just entering a room and finding all of the individuals there sharing your problems and frustrations can change your whole outlook. It can be a totally revealing and very positive experience. RESOLVE is one such organization. (For further information, consult the appendix.)

Once a diagnosis is arrived at one has to sit back and await the results of therapy. After many years of trying to achieve pregnancy, further waiting becomes exceedingly difficult. Nevertheless, just as the year's period of time was necessary to attempt pregnancy before treatment, very often at least this period of time must be allowed to see whether or not therapy will achieve success.

One of the most difficult things to do is to wait. It is especially difficult when other couples around you are having children, most frequently without much difficulty or thought. The feelings are best handled by joining in groups to share in problems and by discussing your feelings openly with your physician. In a certain sense, one has to be able to sit back and allow pregnancy to happen. I am not suggesting that you take the old "vacation cure" but I am attempting to point out that if somehow, after all of these years of effort, while therapy is being instituted, a dispassionate, nonjudgmental attitude could be maintained, the time may be better tolerated. During this period of time you need to have "a place to put your head." There are various ways to diffuse some of the tension and the anxiety of the period. Counseling, consciousness raising sessions, talking to friends and relatives, sharing your feelings, psychotherapy and even Zen exercises, meditation and strenuous exercise all have their roles. Each individual has to find what works for him or her.

Even if it is not possible for a couple to produce a pregnancy, it is still possible for them to have a child. Adoption can result in a child of your own as completely as by almost any other means. Love, environment, guidance, shared experiences, the fulfillment of mutual needs, all contribute to the relationship between child and parent. It becomes immaterial if the child is genetically that of the parents or the result of adoption. Most areas have licensed child-placing agencies which can be helpful in arranging an adoption. In the event that this becomes too difficult because of an excessively long waiting list, occasionally an independent or private adoption through a lawyer or a physician can be arranged. Your local social service agencies and adoption bureaus can be helpful in providing information for your locality and state.

Let me say a word or two about some of the less obvious needs that drive a couple to attempt a pregnancy. Some couples desire pregnancy to hold together a failing marriage. Others consider childbearing the ultimate ego trip in that they see or hope to see little pieces of themselves carried on for future generations to admire. It is presumptious to say that these are insufficient or inappropriate for the treatment of infertility. If such couples were able to have children without medical intervention, no one would be called upon to question the needs and desires of the couple.

Most other couples desire a child to make their lives more complete and to give of themselves to another individual that is uniquely theirs. But, within this group there are also those individuals who desire a pregnancy but not necessarily a child. These are highly motivated individuals who are used to attaining all goals that they have strived for and are used to overcoming barriers by sheer will and determination. Here, they have reached a problem, the inability to conceive, and their natural reaction is to rise to the challenge. The need is not so much a child, but simply the need to succeed and produce a conception. It is very difficult to separate the couples who desire pregnancy, from the couples who desire a child. Indeed, it may be the case that until pregnancy actually occurs, the individuals who desire a pregnancy for the sake of that alone, may not be aware of their feelings. The result is that at times, once pregnancy occurs, instead of feeling elation and joy, these individuals may suddenly find themselves depressed.

The issue becomes more clouded because even couples desiring a child may experience depression and some confusion of emotions with the achieving of a pregnancy. This is because they suddenly realize that there will be changes in their lifestyles, their daily lives, and their means of relating to one another for a very long time. Pregnancy and raising a family represents a very significant change from the status quo.

The point of my discussion is to emphasize that the needs of the individual couple must be constantly re-evaluated throughout the entire diagnostic and therapy period. There is a point when a couple may suddenly find that their original reasons for requesting treatment no longer seem valid, but they may be somewhat ashamed or reluctant to tell their physician. You must understand that it is all right to change your mind at any time. Furthermore, it is important to realize that there are times when the evaluation and therapy of the infertility may be so taxing upon both of you, that the process may become worse than the problem. The "cure" becomes worse than the "disease" when evaluation and therapy begin to invade and negatively affect your private life. At that point it may be appropriate to re-evaluate the situation. You may consider just "walking away" from treatment and come back when and if things feel better. The relationship with your physician must be so close and so sensitive that, paradoxically, you must feel no qualms about stopping treatment at any time. The result is that each visit should be the product of a positive decision. It should not be carried on by rote or the inertia of a workup or therapy plan that has begun. The positive decision must be based on thorough understanding of everything that has been done and everything that will be done. It must be based on the communication between the members of the couple and the treating doctor. If you elect to stop treatment, do not make a decision at that time as to when you will return. If it feels good not to go back, that's fine. If you have a need to return, then that need will express itself in time.

Take things as they come, one thing at a time. Remember, the most complex of knots can be unraveled one step at a time by concentrating and understanding each twist and turn. If each step is understood, slow progress can be tolerated and appreciated and in its own way, even enjoyed. Each minute in time has its own intrinsic beauty and value. It would be unfortunate to overlook it because of an unsatisfying quest. On the other hand, the future holds the answer to most of today's unanswerable questions. The secret is to balance an appreciation of the present with an anticipation of the future.

Glossary

Abortion

The loss of a pregnancy before the fetus can survive on its own.

1. **Spontaneous abortion** – The loss of a pregnancy without any manipulation or the administration of medication to cause the loss of the conception. Also called a miscarriage.

2. **Induced abortion** – The purposeful termination of a pregnancy by the use of instruments or medication.

Adhesion

Scar tissue bands attached to organ surfaces capable of connecting, covering or distorting organs, such as tubes, ovaries and bowel.

Adrenal Glands

Two small glands one on the top of each kidney which produce many of the important steroid hormones including cortisone and a normally small amount of sex hormones.

Adrenogenital Syndrome

A disorder caused by a shift in the hormone production of the adrenal gland frequently resulting in a higher production of male hormones and male secondary sex characteristics in a woman.

Agglutination of Sperm	A sticking together of sperm cells.
Androgens	The general class of male sex hormones. Testosterone is the notable example.
Anovulation	The total absence of ovulation. Note, this is not necessarily the same as "amenorrhea." Menses may still occur with anovulation.
Anovulatory Bleeding	Menses that occur without ovulation. The menstrual pattern is totally random occurring at unpredictable intervals and in irregular amounts varying from spotting to major vaginal bleeding.
Artificial Insemination	The introduction of sperm into a woman's vagina or cervix using instrumentation rather than a penis. 1. **Artificial Insemination – Homologous or Husband (AIH)** – The introduction of a husband's sperm into his wife's vagina or cervix using instruments in order to produce a pregnancy. 2. **Artificial Insemination – Donor (AID)** – The introduction of sperm from an unidentified donor into a woman's vagina or cervix using instruments, in order to produce a pregnancy. 3. **Split Ejaculate Insemination** – Using the first portion of the semen produced by the husband for artificial insemination.
Azospermia	The absence of sperm cells in the semen specimen.
Basal Body Temperature	The temperature of a woman recorded immediately upon awakening before any activity of any kind.

The temperatures are taken orally or rectally and are recorded on a graph. The shape of the curve produced can provide some evidence of ovulation.

Bicornuate Uterus A congenital malformation of the uterus in which it is composed of two smaller horn-shaped bodies each having one Fallopian tube.

Cervix The lowermost portion of the uterus joining it with the vagina. A canal runs through the cervix and is continuous with the cavity of the uterus.

Cilia Microscopic hair-like projections from the surface of a cell capable of beating in a coordinated fashion.

Clomid See Clomiphene Citrate.

Clomiphene Citrate A synthetic drug used to stimulate the hypothalamus and pituitary gland to increase FSH and LH production. It is usually used to treat anovulation but has other uses. This is the generic name for Clomid.

Coitus Intercourse, making love, having sexual relations.

Congenital A non-hereditary characteristic or defect existing since birth.

Conception A pregnancy. Sometimes called a "conceptus."

Contraception Birth control. Using artificial means to prevent pregnancy.

Corpus Luteum A specialized yellow structure that forms on the surface of the ovary at the site of ovulation. It produces the progesterone characteristic of the second half of the cycle and is necessary to prepare the uterine lining for implantation by the fertilized egg.

Cortisol
An important hormone produced by the adrenal glands.

Cryptorchidism
The condition of having testes that have not descended from the abdomen into the scrotum.

Culdoscopy
See Endoscopy.

Dilation and Curettage
An operative procedure where the opening of the uterus, the cervix, is stretched (dilation) and the lining of the uterus scraped (curettage). Sometimes referred to as a D&C.

Dysmenorrhea
Having painful menstruation.

Dyspareunia
Having pain on intercourse.

Ectopic Pregnancy
A pregnancy that grows on a surface other than the cavity of the uterus. In most cases this requires surgery.
1. **Tubal Pregnancy** − A pregnancy that implants in the Fallopian tube.
2. **Ovarian Pregnancy** − A pregnancy that implants on the ovary.
3. **Abdominal Pregnancy** − A pregnancy that implants on the surface of one of the organs in the abdomen other than the tubes or ovaries.

Ejaculation
The release of seminal fluid and sperm from the penis during orgasm.

Endocrine System   A system of ductless glands producing hormones. The system includes the pituitary, parathyroid, thyroid and adrenal glands, the testes and the ovaries.

Endocrinologist   A physician who specializes in the diagnosis and treatment of diseases of the hormone systems.

Endometriosis   A condition where endometrium, the tissue which is normally found lining the uterine cavity, is found on other surfaces. These other surfaces may be the Fallopian tubes, ovaries, the outside of the uterus and/or the surface of the abdominal cavity.

Endometrium   The specialized tissue layer lining the cavity of the uterus.

Endometrial Biopsy   The removal of a small sample of the lining of the uterus for microscopic examination.

Endosalpinx   The specialized tissue lining the Fallopian tube.

Endoscopy   The direct visualization of the inside of the human body by the insertion of a telescope-like device into that part of the body.
　　1. **Culdoscopy** – A minor surgical procedure where a telescope-like device is inserted through a small incision in the back of the vagina in order to visualize the ovaries, Fallopian tubes and uterus. Limited surgery may also be done with this procedure.
　　2. **Laparoscopy** – A minor surgical procedure where a telescope-like device is inserted through a small incision in the umbilicus (the navel) in order to visualize the abdominal con-

tents including the ovaries, Fallopian tubes and the uterus. Limited surgery may also be done with this procedure.

3. **Hysterocopy** – A minor surgical procedure where a telescope-like device is inserted through the cervix into the cavity of the uterus in order to directly visualize the entire cavity. An incision is not needed to insert the telescope.

Epididymis   A coiled tubular structure in the male which receives sperm from the testes. The sperm is stored, nourished and matured for a period of several months, then conducted into the vas deferens.

Erection   The state where the penis, when aroused, is engorged, erect and somewhat rigid.

Estrogen   The primary female hormone. It is a steroid hormone produced mainly by the ovaries from puberty to menopause, and in lesser amounts by the adrenal gland and fatty tissue.

Fallopian Tubes   Paired hollow tubular structures found extending from the body of the uterus toward the ovaries. These structures pick up the egg through their funnel-shaped ends and conduct it to the uterus. Fertilization takes place within this structure. Also called the oviduct.

Fertilization   The union of a sperm and an egg by penetration.

Fetus   The stage of development of an animal or human pregnancy while still in the uterus from the third month until delivery.

Fibroid Tumor	A benign (non-cancerous) tumor found within the wall of the uterus sometimes distorting uterine and/or tubal anatomy. Also known as a myoma.
Fimbria	The fluted funnel-shaped outermost portion of the Fallopian tube specialized in egg pickup.
Follicle	The structure in the ovary that has nurtured the ripening egg and from which the egg is released.
Follicular Stimulating Hormone (FSH)	A hormone produced and released from the pituitary gland. In the female it stimulates estrogen production and development of follicles in the ovary. Follicular stimulation by FSH is necessary for preparation for ovulation. In the male FSH stimulates sperm production.
Frigidity	The inability of a woman to experience sexual arousal.
Genetic	Referring to characteristics transmitted by hereditary.
Genetic Studies	Laboratory studies allowing the identification of certain abnormal states and hereditary disorders. This is usually done by studying certain tissues or white blood cells. The tests are also known as karyotyping.
Gonadotropins	Pituitary hormones, FSH and LH which bio-chemically stimulate the testes or ovaries.
Gonads	A general term referring to the glands which make reproductive cells. The testes in the male and ovaries in the female.

Gonorrhea	A highly contagious disease caused by gonococcus bacteria which affects the male and female reproductive systems. Other organ systems may be involved. The disease is spread mainly through sexual intercourse, and can affect fertility.
Gynecologist	A physician who specializes in the diagnosis and treatment of diseases of the female reproductive system.
Hormone	A chemical produced by a ductless gland of the body.
Hostility Factor	A condition that results in the lack of survival of sperm cells in vaginal or cervical fluids. It manifests itself as a poor post-coital test.
Hühner Test	See Postcoital Test.
Human Chorionic Gonadotropin (HCG)	A hormone produced by the human placenta and which maintains the corpus luteum beyond its usual fourteen day life span. The result is a continual source of progesterone to support an early pregnancy. This hormone may be injected following HMG to trigger ovulation. It is also the basis of most pregnancy tests.
Human Menopausal Gonadotropins (HMG)	The generic name for Pergonal. This is an extract of menopausal urine containing FSH and LH. HMG is administered by injection to treat certain types of anovulation in women and azo- or oligo-spermia in men.
Husband Artificial Insemination	See Artificial Insemination.

194

Hydrosalpinx   A large fluid filled, club-shaped Fallopian tube closed at the fimbriated end (at the end closest to the ovary). It is a cause of infertility.

Hydrotubation   A procedure whereby the Fallopian tubes are "washed" with a sterile solution injected through the cervix. The solution may or may not have medication in it. Its role in the treatment of infertility is controversial. Also known as hydropertubation, pertubation and tubal lavage.

Hymen   A membranous covering at the opening of the vagina. Its thickness may vary from woman to woman. If it is thin enough it will break with her first complete vaginal penetration. If it is quite thick surgical removal may be necessary.

Hypospadius   A malformation of the penis in which the urethral opening, the opening through which urine and sperm leave the penis, is found on the underside rather than at the tip of the penis.

Hypothalamus   The region of the brain just above the pituitary that controls the hormone production and release by the gland.

Hypothyroidism   A state of reduced thyroid function.

Hysterectomy   The surgical removal of the uterus.

Hysteroscopy   See Endoscopy.

Hystero-salpingogram   An x-ray procedure that is done by injecting a fluid which can be seen on x-ray through the cervix into the uterus and tubes. It is frequently performed to see if the Fallopian tubes are open and if the uterine cavity is of normal shape. Also called a Uterotubogram.

Implantation   The adhering of a fertilized egg to the lining of the uterus.

Impotence   The inability of a male to have or maintain an erection of his penis.

In Vitro Fertilization   An experimental procedure in which an egg is removed from a ripe follicle and fertilized by a sperm cell outside the human body. The fertilized egg is allowed to divide in a protected environment for about two days and then is inserted back into the uterus of the woman who produced the egg. (See text for discussion.) Also called "a test tube baby" and "test tube fertilization."

Insufflation of the Tubes   See Rubin Test.

Interstitial Cell   See Leydig Cells.

Infertility   The inability of a heterosexual couple to conceive a pregnancy after one year of regular unprotected intercourse.
    1. **Primary Infertility** – The inability of a couple to conceive after one year of regular unprotected intercourse, with no previous pregnancies having occurred.
    2. **Secondary Infertility** – Infertility occurring after at least one successful pregnancy and delivery.

Karyotype   See Genetic Studies.

196

Klinefelter's Syndrome	A condition in which a male has XXY sex chromosomes instead of XY. A man with this condition is usually sterile.
Laparoscopy	See Endoscopy.
Laparotomy	Abdominal surgery.
Leydig Cells	Cells in the testes that produce testosterone. Also called interstitial cells.
Libido	Sexual desire.
Luteal Phase	The last fourteen days of an ovulatory cycle, associated with progesterone production.
Luteinizing Hormone (LH)	A hormone produced and released by the pituitary gland. In the female it is responsible for ovulation and the maintenance of the corpus luteum for progesterone production. In the male it stimulates testosterone production and is important in spermatogenesis (the production of sperm cells).
Menarche	The age at which a female has her first menstrual flow (period).
Menopause	The time of a woman's last "regular" menstrual flow, and marks the beginning of the failure of the ovary. 1. **Physiologic Menopause** – Menopause occurring spontaneously. The normal cessation of ovarian function usually between age forty-five to fifty. Also known as the "change of life."

2. **Surgical Menopause** – Menopause resulting from the surgical removal of the ovaries.

Menstruation

The regular shedding of the lining of the uterus usually resulting in cyclic monthly vaginal bleeding. This occurs in the absence of pregnancy from menarche to menopause.

Microsurgery

Reconstructive surgery done with the aid of magnification, frequently with a microscope, utilizing extremely fine suture material and very gentle manipulation of the tissue. The result when applied to Fallopian tube or vas deferens surgery appears to be a significant increase in successful reconstruction.

Miscarriage

See Abortion.

Mittleschmertz

Pain felt by some women at mid-cycle during ovulation. It is not absolute proof of ovulation nor is its absence proof that ovulation does not occur.

Morphology of Sperm

The study of the shape of sperm cells. This evaluation is part of a semen analysis.

Motility of Sperm

The ability of sperm cells to move. This evaluation is part of a semen analysis.

Myomectomy

The surgical removal of fibroid tumors from the wall of the uterus.

Nidation

See Implantation.

Obstetrician

A physician who treats pregnant women, provides care for the pregnancy and manages labor and delivery of the baby.

Oligospermia	A scarcity of sperm in a semen sample.
Orchitis	An inflammation of the testes.
Orgasm	The moment of highest sexual excitement. In the male this is marked by ejaculation. In the female this is a time of pleasure with series of muscular contractions of the pelvic muscles.
Ovarian Dysgenesis	See Turner's Syndrome.
Ovaries	The female sex gland with both a reproductive function (releasing eggs) and a hormone function (producing estrogen and progesterone).
Oviduct	The Fallopian tube.
Ovulation	The release of a mature egg from the surface of the ovary.
Ovum	An egg.
Pap Test	A screening test to examine a woman for the presence of cervical cancer. It is done by gently touching a cotton swab on the cervix and then wiping the swab on a slide which is treated and examined under a microscope.
Penis	The male organ used for sexual intercourse and urination.
Pergonal	The brand name under which Human Menopausal Gonadotropin (HMG) is sold.
Peritoneal Cavity	The abdominal cavity.

Peritoneum	The lining of the abdominal cavity.
Peritubal Adhesions	Connective tissue bands around the Fallopian tubes sometimes immobilizing or obstructing the tubes. The result may be a disturbance in egg pickup and infertility.
Pituitary Gland	A gland located at the base of the brain, below the hypothalamus, which controls almost every endocrine gland in the body. It thus controls human growth, development, functioning and reproduction. Also known as the "master gland."
Polycystic Ovary Syndrome	A condition in which a woman has enlarged ovaries containing multiple cysts and a thickened coat on the surface of the ovary. The woman usually ovulates infrequently or not at all. Stein-Leventhal Syndrome is a form of Polycystic Ovary Syndrome.
Postcoital Test	The microscopic study of samples of vaginal and cervical secretions taken several hours after sexual relations. The physician looks for moving, apparently live, sperm cells. Also known as the Sims-Hühner test, the Hühner Test, the P. K. test and the P. C. test.
Progesterone	A hormone produced and released by the corpus luteum of the ovary during the second half of an ovulatory cycle. It is necessary for the preparation of the lining of the uterus for the implantation of the fertilized egg. It is also produced by the placenta during pregnancy.
Prostate Gland	A gland that surrounds the male urethra at its exit from the bladder and contributes secretions to the seminal fluid.

Puberty	The age at which the testes and ovaries begin to function. At this time the young man or woman develops the appropriate sexual characteristics and conception becomes possible.
Retrograde Ejaculation	A condition in which sperm flows backward into the bladder instead of out through the penis during ejaculation.
Retroverted Uterus	A uterus tilted backward toward the woman's back rather than the more common state of tilting toward the front of the abdomen. By itself this should not be a cause of infertility. Also known as a "tilted" or "tipped" uterus.
Rubin Test	A test to demonstrate that the Fallopian tubes are open. Carbon dioxide, a gas, is passed into the uterus and its pressure measured. If the tubes are open the gas will leak out and the pressure will remain low. The woman will also complain of shoulder pain if the tubes are not completely obstructed.
Scrotum	A sac composed mainly of skin found below the penis which holds the testes.
Secondary Infertility	See Infertility.
Semen	The liquid secretions and sperm cells that are released from the penis during ejaculation.
Semen Analysis	The microscopic study of a fresh semen sample. The fluid volume is measured. The number of sperm cells per unit volume is counted and expressed as

millions of cells per cubic centimeter. The percent normally shaped cells, and percent moving cells are also reported.

Septum

An abnormality in organ structure present since birth in which a wall is present where one should not exist.

1. **Septate Uterus** – A uterus with a wall projecting into its cavity.
2. **Vaginal Septum** – A wall present dividing the vagina lengthwise or obstructing it with a side-to-side placement.

Seminiferous Tubules

Structure within the testes that produces sperm cells.

Sims-Hühner Test

See Post-coital Test.

Spermatozoa

Male reproductive cells. Also known as sperm cells.

Spermatogenesis

The production of sperm cells.

Spinnbarkeit

The stretchability of cervical mucus. This is a rough measure of how easily sperm cells can enter and penetrate the cervical secretions.

Stein-Leventhal Disease

See Polycystic Ovary Syndrome.

Testicle

See Testis.

Testis

The male sex gland with both a reproductive function (producing sperm cells) and a hormone function (producing testosterone).

Testicular Biopsy   A minor surgical procedure in which a small piece of a testis is removed for microscopic study. This is usually reserved for a male who has extremely low or absent sperm production.

Testosterone   A steroid hormone, made by the testes, which is the most potent male sex hormone.

Thyroid Gland   A gland in the neck which produces thyroid hormone.

Thyroxin   One of the hormones of the thyroid gland.

"Tipped" Uterus   See Retroverted Uterus.

Tubal Insufflation   See Rubin Test.

Turner's Syndrome   An abnormality of genetic material in which a female has XO sex chromosomes instead of the normal XX. Most women with this condition are sterile.

Urethra   The passage within the penis which carries, at different times, urine and semen.

Urologist   A physician who diagnoses and treats diseases of the male or female urinary tract and treats problems of the male reproductive tract.

Uterus   A hollow, muscular structure which is part of the female reproductive tract that is the source of a woman's menses. Its prime reproductive function is to house, protect and nourish the developing fetus.

Vagina   A tubular passageway in the female connecting the external sex organs with the cervix and uterus. Also known as the "birth canal."

Vaginismus
A condition in which there is an extreme constricture of the muscles about the opening of the vagina, making the insertion of a penis during sexual relations painful, difficult or impossible.

Varicocele
A varicose vein around the vas deferens and the testis. This may be a cause of male infertility.

Varicocelectomy
A surgical procedure for the correction of a varicocele.

Vas Deferens
A thick walled tubular structure running from each testis into the ejaculatory duct. These structures carry sperm from the epididymis to the penis.

Vasectomy
A minor surgical procedure done to interrupt and obstruct the vas deferens. This is done as a male sterilization procedure.

Appendix I

Numbers and Normals

I. Statistics

    A. *50–60%* of couples of reproductive age who present for an adequate infertility evaluation conceive with therapy

    5% of infertile couples become pregnant without therapy

    B. The following are pregnancy rates of sexually active women of childbearing age:

    after one month of sexual relations – 25% will be pregnant

    after six months – 63% will be pregnant

    after nine months –75% will be pregnant

    after twelve months – 80% will be pregnant

    after eighteen months – 90% will be pregnant

    C. 15% of couples of reproductive age in the United States are infertile. That is approximately one couple in six. The actual number is in excess of ten million people.

    D. Causes of Infertility

    40% – male factor

    50% – female factor

15% anovulation
30% tubal problem
5% cervical problem
10% – no cause can be found. (Note that in a recent study the percentage of unexplained infertility was reduced to 3.5%.)

E. Greater than 90% of patients who are completely evaluated will have a cause found for their infertility. 50–60% will conceive.

F. 95% of women who are anovulatory will be made to ovulate by medical treatment. About 50% will conceive.

II. Normal values for a semen analysis – in our laboratory count – greater than twenty million cells/ml. with a mean of 40–80 million cells/ml. Volume – 2–5 ml.
Motility at two hours – greater than 60%
Morphology – greater than 60% normal forms
Fructose – (+)
Note that the sperm count may vary in the same patient from ejaculate to ejaculate by 20%. Furthermore, even counting the same specimen several times may be associated with an error of 10%.

HYSTEROSALPINGOGRAM

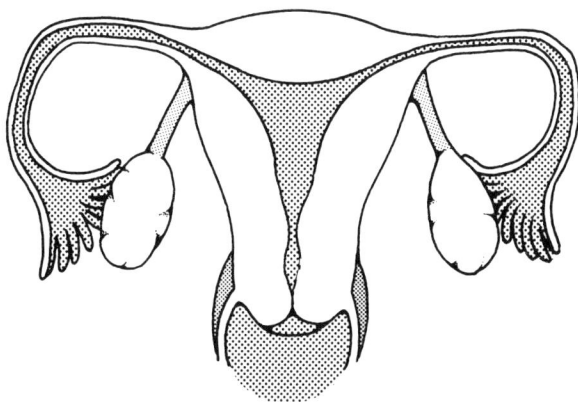

anatomy

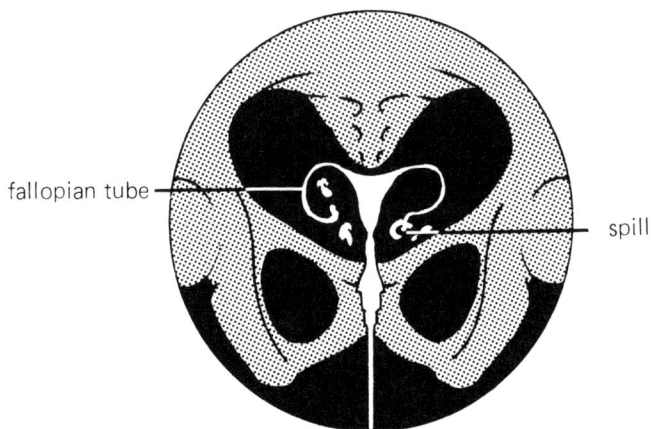

fallopian tube

spill

x-ray

NORMAL

septum dividing
the uterine cavity

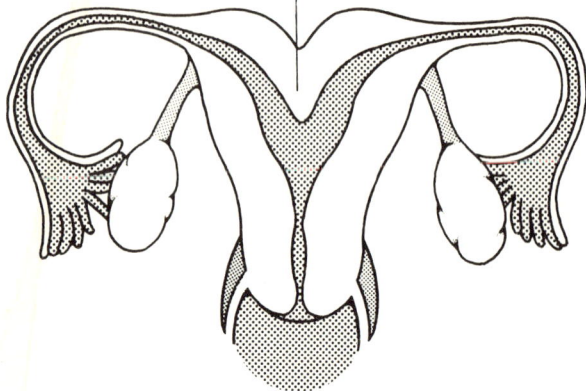

anatomy

divide of cavity
of uterus

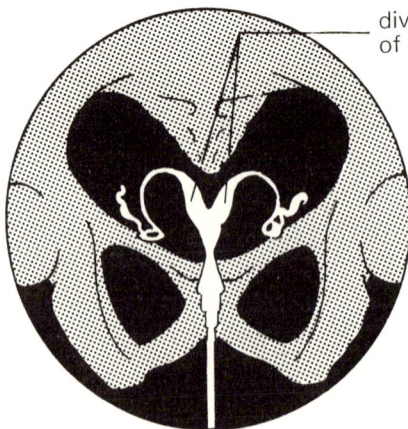

x-ray

SEPTUM

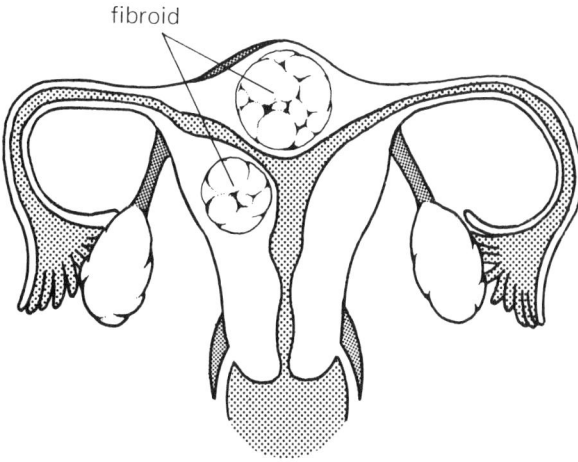

fibroid

anatomy

fibroid outlined on
hysterosalpingogram

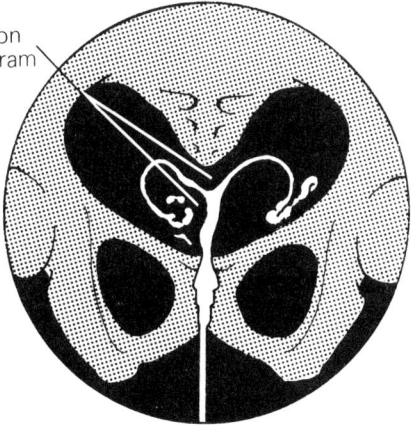

x-ray

FIBROID

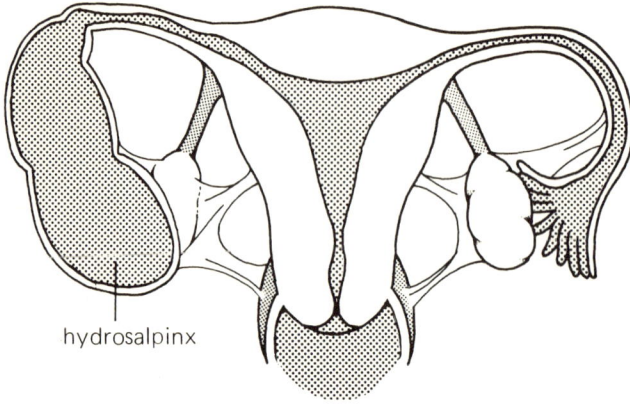

hydrosalpinx

anatomy

hydrosalpinx—an
obstructed sac-like
tube

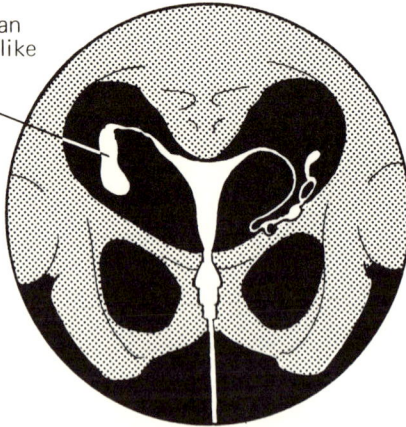

x-ray

HYDROSALPINX

Changes in plasma progesterone during cycle

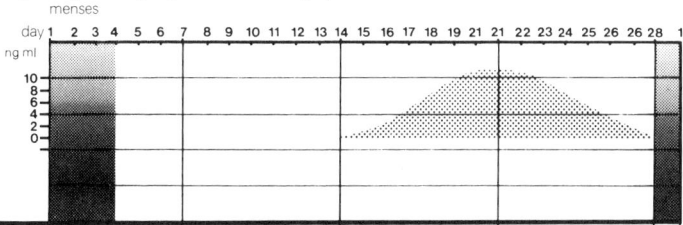

menses

| day | 1 | 2 | 3 | 4 | 5 | 6 | 7 | 8 | 9 | 10 | 11 | 12 | 13 | 14 | 15 | 16 | 17 | 18 | 19 | 21 | 21 | 22 | 23 | 24 | 25 | 26 | 26 | 28 | 1 |

ng ml

10
8
6
4
2
0

Changes in basal body temperature during cycle

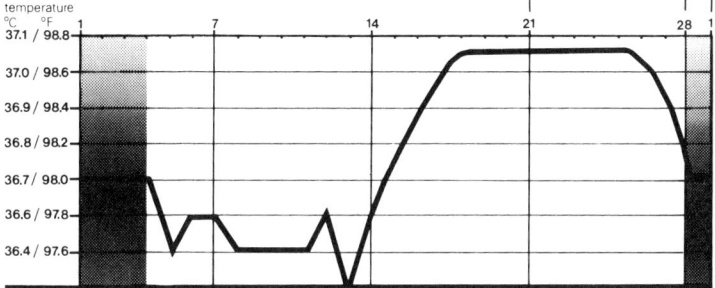

temperature

°C / °F

| 1 | 7 | 14 | 21 | 28 | 1 |

37.1 / 98.8
37.0 / 98.6
36.9 / 98.4
36.8 / 98.2
36.7 / 98.0
36.6 / 97.8
36.4 / 97.6

Changes in endometrium during cycle

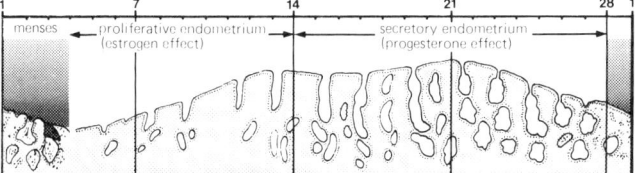

| 1 | 7 | 14 | 21 | 28 | 1 |

menses | proliferative endometrium (estrogen effect) | secretory endometrium (progesterone effect)

Changes in cervical mucus during cycle

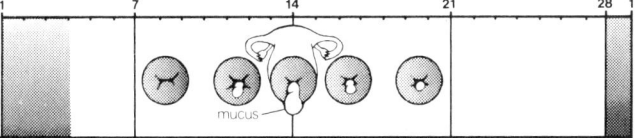

| 1 | 7 | 14 | 21 | 28 | 1 |

mucus

Timing of infertility tests

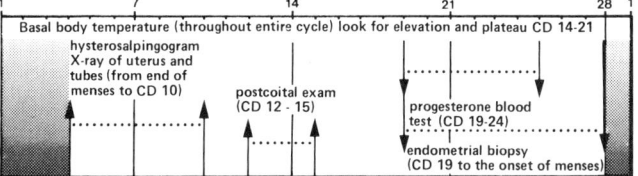

| 1 | 7 | 14 | 21 | 28 | 1 |

Basal body temperature (throughout entire cycle) look for elevation and plateau CD 14-21

hysterosalpingogram
X-ray of uterus and
tubes (from end of
menses to CD 10)

postcoital exam
(CD 12 - 15)

progesterone blood
test (CD 19-24)

endometrial biopsy
(CD 19 to the onset of menses)

211

Appendix II

For Further Information

I. Books
1. S. J. Behrman, and Robert W. Kistner, *Progress in Infertility* (Boston: Little Brown and Company, 1975) – an excellent medical textbook discussing male and female infertility, diagnosis and treatment.
2. Richard D. Amelar, and Lawrence Dubin and Patrick C. Walsh, *Male Infertility* (W. B. Saunders Company Philadelphia 1977) – an excellent medical textbook confined to male infertility.
3. Leon Speroff, Robert H. Glass, and Nathan G. Kase, *Clinical Gynecologic Endocrinology and Infertility* (The Williams and Wilkins Company, Baltimore, 1978) – an excellent medical textbook discussing the female hormonal system and infertility in general.
4. *Woman's Body – An Owner's Manual* (Paddington Press Ltd., London, 1977) – a very complete book describing in ordinary language all aspects of the female body and its functioning.
5. *Man's Body – An Owner's Manual* (Paddington Press Ltd., London, 1977) –

a complete description of the male body and in its workings in ordinary language.

II. JOURNALS

1. *Fertility and Sterility* – a monthly medical journal published by the American Fertility Society. This publication presents the latest in research within the field of the Reproductive Sciences.
2. Other medical journals for the specialists of Urology, Obstetrics and Gynecology, and Endocrinology can be provided at the library of your nearest medical school or college. The librarian can be of assistance.

III. ORGANIZATIONS

A. THE UNITED STATES

1. American Fertility Society
1608 13th Avenue, South
Suite 101
Birmingham, Alabama 35205
This organization can act as a source of specialists from which you may choose a specialist in infertility.
2. Planned Parenthood Federation of America
810 Seventh Avenue
New York, N.Y. 10019
This organization can act as a source of information about reproductive problems in general and may be able to provide specific information about health care in various communities.
3. RESOLVE, Inc.
P.O. Box 474
Belmont, Massachusetts 02178

A nonprofit organization completely
directed toward the help and support of
the infertile couple. Counseling, support
groups, medical information and a local
referral service are only part of its work.

B. THE UNITED KINGDOM
1. British Fertility Society
   Chairman: Dr. Patrick Steptoe, Oldham
   General Hospital
   Secretary: Mr. Victor Lewis, Watford
   General Hospital
   Concerned with research on human
   reproduction and particularly in relation to
   fertility and sterility problems.
2. Family Planning Association Information
   Service
   27 Mortimer Street
   London W1.
   Offers information service on all aspects of
   family planning and refers patients to
   NHS-run Family Planning Clinics. Some
   of these incorporate a separate Infertility
   Clinic. FPA Information Service also refers
   patients to hospital specialists.
3. National Association for the Childless
   318 Summer Lane
   Birmingham.
   B19 3RL
   General counseling and advice about fertility
   testing, nearest fertility clinics, hospital
   specialists, etc. Also offers moral support
   to couples.
   Operates as project of Birmingham Settlement
   – a government-sponsored social worker

organization – which underwrites costs of N.A.C. Has applied for registration as charity.

C. AUSTRALIA AND CANADA

1. The many Family Planning Association offices in Canada and Australia provide information and advice concerning fertility problems, as well as their general help with all aspects of family planning.

Index

gonorrhea, 60, 70, 72, 92, 194

H

HCG, see Human Chorionic
Gonadotropin
heat, reducing sperm production, 63,
92–3
HMG, see Human Menopausal
Gonadotropin
hormones, 194
  and abortion, 69–70
  action on uterus, 35–6
  causing habitual abortion, 166
  controlling ovulation, 33–5; 36, 37
  deficiency, 65–8, 69–70
  female, 27
  hormone analogues, 179
  male, 19, 61–2
  tests, 98
  treatment of deficiency, 130–1,
  132–41
  treatment of habitual abortion, 169–70
hostility factor, 83–5, 124, 126, 194
Hühner Test, 202
Human Chorionic Gonadotropin
  (HCG), 130, 131, 133, 138–9,
  140, 155, 159–60, 194
Human Menopausal Gonadotropin
  (HMG), 130, 133, 139–40, 155, 194
hydrosalpinx, 195; 71, 112, 152
hydrotubation, 195
hymen, 22, 142, 195
hypospadias, 58–9, 195
hypothalamus, 33, 65, 66–9, 134–5, 139,
  179, 195; 64–7
hypothyroidism, 195
hysterectomy, 195

hysterosalpingogram, 78, 106, 108–15,
  118, 142, 143, 167–8, 170, 195–6; 109,
  111–14, 127
hysteroscopy, 78, 116–18, 142, 143,
  168, 170, 192; 117

I

implantation, 32–3, 35–6, 196
impotence, 196
in vitro fertilization, 174–6, 196
infertility, causes, 54–89
  definition, 14–15, 27–8, 196
  female, 53, 63–81
  male, 53, 55–63
  myths, 43–53
  primary, 16, 196; secondary, 16, 196
  spontaneous fertility rate, 52
  tests, 90–128; 127
  treatment, 129–61
intrauterine contraceptives (IUD), 73,
  118

J

jogging, effect on ovulation, 158–60

K

Kallman's Syndrome, 61–2
karyotyping, 166
Klinefelter's Syndrome, 60–1, 197

L

labia majora, 21
labia minora, 21

219

laparoscopy, 116, 119–21, 142, 146,
  153, 191–2; *120, 147*
laparotomy, 197
leiomyoma, 78
Leydig cells, 197
LH, *see* luteinizing hormone
libido, 197
lubricants, 93
luteal phase, 197
luteal phase defect, 70
luteinizing hormone (LH), 197
  deficiency of, 61–2, 63, 139–40
  and failure of ovulation, 64–8
  64–7
  production of, 33; *36, 37*
  tests, 98
  treatment of deficiency, 130, 134–5
  136, 179
lysis of adhesions, 146; *147, 148*

M

male anatomy, 17–21; *18*
male factor infertility, 53, 55–63
  evaluation, 95–8
  treatment, 130–2
male-female interaction, 81–8
  infertility tests, 123–6
  see also sexual intercourse
medroxyprogesterone, 151–2
menarche, 197
menopause, 139, 197–8
menstruation, 24, 36–7, 198
  anovulatory bleeding, 45–6, 91,
    188
  cramps, 91–2
  effect of stress on, 86
  menstrual cycle, 24, 38–41; *39, 40*

painless, 91
microsurgery, 132, 148–50, 173, 198
miscarriage, *see* abortion
mittleschmerz, 92, 198
morphology, sperm, 198
motility, sperm, 198
mumps, 60, 92
myoma, *see* fibroids
myomectomy, 143, 170, 198; *144*

O

oligospermia, 199
orchitis, 60, 199
orgasm, 20, 199
ovaries, 199, adhesions, 72, 76
  corpus luteum, 35–6
  cysts, 72, 153, 154–5
  endometriosis, 74
  failure of, 63–5, 67
  hormone stimulation, 33; *36, 37*
  hyper-stimulation syndrome, 140
  ovarian pregnancy, 190
  polycystic ovary syndrome, 154–5,
    200
  structure and formation, 21, 24, 27,
    30
  transplants, 174–5
  wedge resection, 155; *156*
  see also ovulation
oviducts, *see* Fallopian tubes
ovulation, 27, 30, 32–5, 44–5, 199;
  31, 36, 37
  cramp associated with, 91–2
  effect of stress on, 86
  effect on cervical mucus, 24
  effected by physical exercise, 158–60
  failure of, 29, 63–9; *64–7*

occurrence in menstrual cycle, 38, 41
postpill amenorrhea, 160–71
tests, 98–106; *100*
treatment to produce, 133–6, 137–41,
    172
ovum, blighted pregnancy, 164–5
fertilization, 30, 32, 41–2, 43–4
genetic abnormalities, 87–8
in vitro fertilization, 176–8, 196
production of, 27, 30, 33

P

pan-hypopituitarism, 62
Pap test, 199
P.C. test, *see* post-coital tests
pelvic adhesions, 49
pelvic infections, 70–3, 92
penis, 199
    abnormalities, 58–9, 82, 97; *59*
    structure and function, 17–20; *18*
Pergonal, 130, 131, 133, 134, 139–41,
    155, 199
periods, *see* menstruation
peritoneum, 200
peritubal adhesions, *see* adhesions
physical exercise, effect on ovulation,
    158–60
pituitary gland, FSH and LH deficiency,
    61–2, 65–6, 68; *65–7*
    function of, 33, 35, 200; *36, 37, 64*
    treatment of hormone deficiency,
        130, 134–5, 139–40
P.K. test, 200
placenta, 32, 36
polycystic ovary syndrome, 154–5,
    200
polyps, 110, 116, 118

post-coital tests, 81, 84, 123–5, 200;
    127
pregnancy, 30–42
    abnormalities, 46–7
    blighted, 164–5, 171
    ectopic, 190
    multiple, 134, 140
    tubal, 151, 172–3, 190
    see also fertilization
Pregnyl, 133
primary infertility, 16
progesterone, and basal body
        temperature, 98–101
    function of, 35–6, 200
    and habitual abortion, 166, 169–70
    influence on secretory endometrium,
        38, 101
    lack of as cause of miscarriage,
        69–70
    production of, 27, 35
    tests for deficiency, 104–6, 132–3,
        137–8; *105, 127*
    treatment for deficiency, 136–7
    use in diagnosing cause of
        infertility, 68
Prolactin, 141
prostate gland, 19, 20, 200
Provera, 153–4
psychological problems, 85–7
puberty, 201

R

radiation, damage to sperm production,
    63
rectal intercourse, 82–3
retrograde ejaculation, 20, 58, 63, 201

221